Acclaim for

THE OVERNIGHT DIET

"The ultimate blueprint for anyone trying to lose weight. This one-of-a-kind diet delivers exactly what dieters are desperately looking for: an easy-to-follow plan for significant rapid weight loss that lasts while also promoting better health, fighting disease, and increasing longevity. And it's the first diet book that gives dieters that extra edge in the battle of the bulge by maintaining lean muscle mass."

—Louis J. Aronne, MD, clinical professor of medicine, Weill Cornell Medical College/New York-Presbyterian Hospital, and *New York Times* bestselling author of *The Skinny*

"Caroline Apovian knows how to make the science of weight loss entertaining and has created a diet that works on the inside for results on the outside!"

—Cynthia Stamper Graff, author of *Lean for Life*

"THE OVERNIGHT DIET is anything but your standard fare in diet books. It's the real thing for people who are serious about losing weight as quickly as possible in a healthy, long-lasting way."

—George L. Blackburn, MD, PhD, associate director of nutrition and the S. Daniel Abraham chair in nutrition medicine at Harvard Medical School

THE OVERNIGHT DIET

THE PROVEN PLAN FOR FAST, PERMANENT WEIGHT LOSS

By CAROLINE APOVIAN, MD

with FRANCES SHARPE,

and in consultation with
Diana Cullum-Dugan, RD
and
Wayne Westcott, PhD

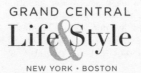

GRAND CENTRAL
Life & Style

NEW YORK · BOSTON

Copyright © 2013 by Caroline Apovian and The Philip Lief Group Inc.

Produced by The Philip Lief Group Inc.

Illustrations by Joung Park

Physicians Protein Smoothies™ is the trademark of Caroline Apovian, MD, and The Philip Lief Group, Inc.

Grand Central Life & Style
Hachette Book Group
237 Park Avenue
New York, NY 10017

www.GrandCentralLifeandStyle.com

Printed in the United States of America

RRD-C

Originally published in hardcover by Hachette Book Group, Inc.

First trade edition: May 2014
10 9 8 7 6 5 4 3 2 1

Grand Central Life & Style is an imprint of Grand Central Publishing.
The Grand Central Life & Style name and logo are trademarks of Hachette Book Group, Inc.

The Hachette Speakers Bureau provides a wide range of authors for speaking events. To find out more, go to www.hachettespeakersbureau.com or call (866) 376-6591.

The publisher is not responsible for websites (or their content) that are not owned by the publisher.

The Library of Congress has cataloged the hardcover edition as follows
Apovian, Caroline M.
  The overnight diet : the proven plan for fast, permanent weight loss / by Caroline Apovian, M.D. ; with Frances Sharpe, Diana Cullum-Dugan RD, and Wayne Westcott, PhD. — First edition.
     pages cm
  Summary: "THE OVERNIGHT DIET is the world's first high-octane hybrid diet designed to produce instant, lasting results, preserve lean muscle, prevent disease, and increase longevity. Now Dr. Caroline Apovian, leading expert and authority on nutrition and weight management, explains the seven-day plan that prevents "Shrinking Muscle Syndrome" and increases lean muscle mass to keep metabolism revved up. The 1-Day Power Up jump-starts fat burning and weight-loss in one night, then the 6-Day Fuel Up keeps the body in fat-burning mode while offering readers a bounty of tasty food options, including peanut butter, avocado, and even chocolate! After losing up to two pounds overnight and up to nine pounds in the first week, the cycle can be repeated every seven days to achieve lightning-fast weight loss, burn fat, reduce water retention and bloating, stave off hunger pangs, and prevent plateaus. This is the ultimate blueprint for anyone who wants to slim down, whether they want to lose five pounds or 50 pounds!"—Provided by publisher.
  ISBN 978-1-4555-1691-9 (hardback) — ISBN 978-1-4555-1692-6 (ebook) — ISBN 978-1-61969-639-6 (audiobook) 1. Weight loss. 2. Reducing diets—Recipes. I. Title.
  RM222.2.A662 2013
  613.2'5—dc23

                                                    2012045480

ISBN 978-1-4555-1693-3 (pbk.)

To my mother, Ines Chinni Apovian,
who has always been ahead of her time.

Acknowledgments

This book could not have been written without the help and dedication of a team of people around me sharing their expertise to create the Overnight Diet. Thank you to Frances Sharpe, and her ability to put it all together; to Diana Cullum-Dugan, whose creative ideas and recipes have no rival; to Wayne Westcott, whose enthusiasm for health and wellness is infectious; to Rita LaRosa Loud, who makes it all happen in the fitness world. Thank you to photographer Thomas Huynh, who worked closely with Wayne Westcott and Rita LaRosa Loud to capture the fitness moves so eloquently. Thank you to illustrator Joung Park, who then transformed those photographs into the beautiful and simple easy-to-follow illustrations you see in this book.

A big thank-you to the team at Grand Central Publishing, especially Diana Baroni and Amanda Englander, both there 24/7 and ready to offer a solution for every little thing.

Thank you to David Blackburn and Rod Egger, who invited the Overnight Diet program into their realm because the philosophy was so closely aligned, and now we have the Physicians Protein Smoothies, Base and Flavor lines. Thank you to George Blackburn, my mentor and now a dear friend, who always steered me the right way, and sees above everyone else.

And a special thank-you to Philip Lief, the other person who also sees above everyone else!

Thank you to my father, Dr. John Apovian, for believing in me, always. And last but not least, thank you to my little family, the Baker boys, Gus, John, and Philip, for supporting me no matter what.

Contents

Part IV.
THE OVERNIGHT DIET FOR LIFE!

THE OVERNIGHT DIET

Introduction

Overnight results *that last*—that's what you get with the Overnight Diet. And it's a big part of how, in the past twenty-plus years, I've helped my patients lose over 1 million pounds. You see, helping people slim down is what I do. I'm not a cardiologist, or a family physician, or an emergency room doctor who dabbles in weight management on the side. I'm an obesity medicine physician, which means that I specialize in weight loss. As the director of the Nutrition and Weight Management Center at Boston Medical Center, I've helped thousands of people just like you quickly and safely lose pounds and inches for good. And as one of the world's leading researchers on obesity and weight loss, I'm privy to—and sometimes I'm the one presenting—the most up-to-the-minute scientific findings on what makes people fat, what keeps them fat, and what works to help them lose that fat forever. In fact, my research colleagues have made a revolutionary scientific discovery that shows why most popular diets are doomed to fail. It's because they lead to muscle wasting, a condition known in medical circles as *sarcopenia*, which sabotages efforts to lose weight. We'll get to the details on that later. For now, just know that I am here to help translate this research and use it to help you lose weight and keep it off.

The Dark Ages of Dieting

Dieting has gotten stuck in the Dark Ages. I pay attention to every diet that comes out because my patients have usually tried them all and failed. It's no wonder. Most are either rehashing the same advice or introducing wacky concepts that aren't based on any research at all. That's why, despite your best efforts, you haven't been able to lose those stubborn pounds. Or maybe you have lost weight but can't seem to keep it from creeping back onto your thighs, butt, and belly, leading to a lifetime of yo-yo dieting. Or perhaps you're a few pounds lighter but still feel and look a bit flabby and, well, marshmallowy. Is that what you want after all that hard work—a jiggly midsection?

You probably feel frustrated and discouraged. I don't blame you. I've been there myself. I know from personal experience just how hard it can be to lose weight with most diets. When I was in college, I gained the "Freshman 10" then went on to achieve the "Sophomore 15" and the "Junior 20" before slimming down and shaping up with what became the Overnight Diet. I listen with great empathy as my patients tell me all the reasons why they haven't succeeded at dieting. For example, Tina, twenty-seven, lamented that one low-calorie diet left her feeling hungry all the time. Jenna, a forty-three-year-old mother of two, complained that she would lose a few pounds then see her weight loss come to a grinding halt even though she was practically starving herself. And fifty-one-year-old Roger told me he would get beyond bored eating the same few bland foods on a diet's "approved" list. The result? They all quit and went right back to their old eating habits. They each told me that they felt like a failure. But I reassured each of them that they hadn't failed dieting; the Dark Ages diets had failed them.

It's bad enough when these diets can't help you reach your goal weight. But for some of my patients, trying to shed pounds with popular diets has had far more dangerous consequences. I've had patients develop high blood pressure, high cholesterol, type 2 diabetes, gout, excruciatingly painful kidney stones, or see their muscles wither away—all from trying to lose weight and get healthy. It doesn't make any sense!

I have news for you. Losing weight shouldn't make you suffer. Slimming down—when you do it the right way with a bounty of nutritious foods—should enhance your health and well-being and make you *feel better, not worse*! Hearing what other diets were doing to my patients infuriated me. Seeing that so many of them were not only *not losing weight* with existing diet plans, but also harming their health, feeling deprived, and feeling depressed, I knew I had to do something about it.

Developing the Next Generation of Dieting

After witnessing the struggles of my patients, it became my mission to engineer a twenty-first-century science-based diet that would help you safely achieve rapid weight loss that lasts. The Overnight Diet is that plan: a revolutionary diet based on nearly twenty-five years of research as well as testing with thousands of everyday people just like you. It takes dieting to a whole new level with real, road-tested benefits.

The Overnight Diet is very simple, but before I give you the ABCs of the program, I want to let you know how I developed it. Here's why: Your health and safety are of the utmost importance to me—and they should be to you, too—so I want you to understand that this isn't some fad diet to lose a few pounds at the expense of your health. Rather, it's backed by decades of scientific research showing that in addition to producing quick results, it promotes better health and even longevity. That's right—it's your ticket to looking better, feeling better, and living longer.

For years in my clinic and at the lab at the Nutrition and Weight Management Center at Boston Medical Center, I had been using two time-tested rapid-weight-loss strategies with great success:

The first came from Dr. George Blackburn and Dr. Bruce Bistrian, the renowned creators of the nation's most respected and widely used medically supervised rapid-weight-loss diet. After my residency in internal medicine, I completed a two-year nutrition and metabolism fellowship with these revered nutrition pioneers and soaked up as much knowledge as I possibly could. Their diet was developed to be used in a highly monitored setting, i.e., the hospital. As successful as it was, I knew that it could be even more accessible and therefore more effective. Over the years, I refined and improved their diet, taking it light-years beyond what they had ever imagined. I have modified it so that it is easier to use and so that you get to eat more food, which allows you to get the lasting results you want with no doctor supervision necessary.

The second is based on a simple dietary habit that has been the subject of decades of research showing that it produces overnight weight loss and a health boost so powerful it increases longevity. It's something humans have been doing for thousands of years. In fact, scientific evidence shows that it's something our bodies are *genetically programmed* to do. But most Americans no longer engage in this once-common practice, and research shows that because of this, our genetic programming has started working against us by piling more and more fat onto our bodies. It's hard to believe, but the weight-loss aspect of this practice has not been explored effectively... until now. I have given this long-standing approach a modern-day reinvention to maximize its flab-fighting ability in the minimum amount of time. The result? Losing more fat faster.

Both strategies had helped my patients knock off unwanted pounds, but I knew they could do even more. One day, one of the staff members at my practice drove up in her new hybrid car, and she started raving about the incredible mileage it got from the combined battery and gas engine. Right then, the wheels in my head started turning, and I had an *aha!* moment.

What if I combined these two separate slim-down strategies into one turbocharged, high-performance diet?

I immediately went to work developing the optimal blend of the best of both plans so they would work synergistically—fueling each other similarly to the way a hybrid car's battery and gas engine work together—to maximize results. I spent years testing and refining this combo diet with real-life people and found that it not only speeds weight loss, but also shatters the typical obstacles to long-term success, making it the ultimate plateau buster. Finally! The next generation of weight loss is here now. So say good-bye to the Dark Ages of dieting and hello to the world's first-ever hybrid diet designed to produce overnight results that last.

Adding Even More Muscle to the Overnight Diet

The synergy that arises from two diet strategies working in tandem is only part of what makes the Overnight Diet so different from any other diet you've tried. Through research, I've also pinpointed the main culprit that thwarts efforts to fight fat, slows metabolism, leads to yo-yo dieting, and can devastate health. And contrary to popular belief, it has nothing to do with a lack of willpower.

It's muscle wasting, a condition known in "doctor speak" as *sarcopenia*, but which I prefer to call the "Shrinking Muscle Syndrome." It is the loss of muscle mass, strength, and function that may occur naturally with age, but that may also occur as a dangerous side effect of or be expedited by most popular weight-loss methods. The nutritional makeup of many diets can cause the body to rob your muscles for energy, leaving you thinner, but weaker and flabbier. Losing muscle from these diets explains why even though your scale may show that "magic number," you still can't fit into your skinny jeans and don't want to wear a bikini because you look flabby and out of shape. But it gets even worse.

If you regain the weight you lost, as an alarming 95 percent of people on Dark Ages diets do according to statistics, you need to know that it typically comes back as fat rather than as muscle, so there's *even more* blubber than before. Losing and regaining weight over and over and over throughout your lifetime can be especially harmful. Eventually a person can balloon up like the Michelin Man and not have enough muscle to support all that weight. Think of trying to hold up a watermelon with a couple of toothpicks—you get the idea. It's what scientists call *sarcopenic obesity*, or fat frail, and it's a scary condition that makes it difficult for people to stand up or even get out of a chair without assistance. Imagine needing help just to go to the bathroom or answer your front door—that's how debilitating it can be.

If our diets and weight-loss methods don't change, in ten years many more people will be in wheelchairs than ever anticipated. Most people who are trying to lose weight have no clue that they could be in danger of developing this condition, but I guarantee that they'll be hearing a lot more about the Shrinking Muscle Syndrome in the coming months and years.

Preventing it is the ultimate key to rapid weight loss that lasts, and it's why I've engineered the Overnight Diet specifically to maintain lean muscle while torching flab. Don't worry, this doesn't mean you have to become a bodybuilder or turn into the Incredible Hulk—in fact, you don't even have to lift a single barbell. What I'm talking about are long, lean, strong muscles that make you look toned and fit. Isn't that what we all want? Just imagine how great it will feel to wave good-bye to someone and not feel that embarrassing arm flab flapping in the breeze.

Look Better, Feel Better, Live Longer

There's more good news—every aspect of the Overnight Diet is designed to promote health and well-being. And I'm not just talking about long-term health benefits that you won't notice until you're in your Golden Years. You'll be thrilled to know that eating the good-for-you foods on this diet can have effects that enhance your health now. Look at what can happen during the first week alone:

- **Immediately:** Compared to eating a fatty breakfast such as greasy bacon or buttery croissants, eating a breakfast such as the ones recommended on the Overnight Diet provides a better boost in mental alertness—no more need for that third cup of coffee to try to power through those morning meetings at work.
- **Within 90 minutes:** Starting just 90 minutes after eating a breakfast similar to what you'll be eating on the Overnight

Diet rather than having a muffin, a scone, or those leftover doughnuts in the break room, the levels of the hunger hormone ghrelin are reduced and remain lowered for three hours. That helps keep your stomach from rumbling.

- **After 24 hours:** You'll lose up to 2 pounds overnight as your body flushes out excess water weight, which reduces insulin levels, improves insulin sensitivity, and minimizes bloat. Plus, it activates the fat-incinerating process.

- **By Day 2:** Eating adequate protein throughout the day as you'll be doing on this diet helps knock out those afternoon energy crashes so you can power through your day.

- **By Night 2:** Eating plentiful amounts of what I call "lean carbs" boosts serotonin production in the brain and can enhance your moods and promote better sleep. Imagine waking up raring to go. Plus, when you sleep better, it helps balance your appetite hormones to control hunger, as well as reducing stress, reducing cravings, and boosting energy.

- **After 1 week:** You could lose up to 9 pounds in one week. In addition, you'll experience reduced hunger, fewer cravings, better moods, higher energy levels, more restful sleep, and enhanced mental alertness. Higher energy levels pump up your desire to get moving with physical activity, which boosts production of a metabolic enzyme called AMPkinase. In turn, this enzyme gives your energy levels an added boost, and it increases production of a hormone called irisin that helps you burn more calories.

Is the Overnight Diet for Me?

Whether you want to lose 5 pounds, 15 pounds, or 50-plus pounds, this hybrid diet will help you do it quickly and safely without feeling deprived. Even if you just want to drop those few extra pounds you piled on over the holidays, you can do it by following this no-fuss plan. In fact, reaching your weight-loss goal has never been so easy. With the Overnight Diet, you can:

- Lose up to 2 pounds overnight and up to 9 pounds the first week, and every week thereafter, until you reach your goal weight.
- Prevent weight-loss plateaus.
- Burn *more* fat faster.
- Eat *more* food while losing *more* weight.
- Exercise *less* while burning *more* fat.
- Stave off hunger pangs.
- Enhance your health.

I've seen it work for thousands of my patients, and I want to see it work for you, too. That's why I'm sharing this program with you in this book. I want you to be able to experience what it feels like to get the rapid results you're looking for and feel good while doing it.

Let's get started!

PART I

HOW THE OVERNIGHT DIET WORKS

CHAPTER 1

Overnight Results That Last

With the Overnight Diet, you get the benefit of not just one, but two diet strategies blended into one hybrid plan. Together, they give you the quick results you want—losing up to 2 pounds overnight and up to 9 pounds in the first week—and help you keep the pounds coming off and staying off so you can finally enjoy a long-term relationship with that sleek new shape of yours. Scientific research shows how each piece of this combo diet primes the body to respond better to the other, creating the optimal physiological conditions for rapid weight loss that lasts.

Tales of the Measuring Tape

"A lot of diets promise fast weight loss, but I couldn't believe it when I lost 2 pounds after the very first day."
—Renée, 32, lost 18 pounds and 3 inches off her waist

Thanks to this synergy, the Overnight Diet safely delivers rapid weight loss, burns more fat, turns off your "fat" genes, reduces water retention and bloating, staves off hunger pangs, and prevents plateaus. And all of that adds up to enhanced motivation. Of course, it's pretty easy to stay motivated when the number on the scale keeps going down and your waistline keeps shrinking week after week.

How does this combo diet get you slim fast? It starts with the 1-Day Power Up, which is based on a dietary habit that humans have been doing for thousands of years—taking a temporary break from solid food. This age-old practice has been reengineered for the twenty-first century to jump-start fat burning and weight loss overnight, while reducing hunger. That's followed by the 6-Day Fuel Up, which builds on the Protein Sparing Modified Fast created by Dr. Blackburn and Dr. Bistrian. "Protein sparing" means that it preserves lean muscle mass, which you'll learn much more about throughout this book. The Protein Sparing Modified Fast has been reformulated to keep the body in fat-burning mode while allowing you to eat a bounty of tasty foods you love, including peanut butter, avocado, and yes, even potatoes. Then you start the 7-day cycle all over again back at the 1-Day Power Up, which reboots your fat-burning engine and promotes overnight weight loss week in and week out. Just keep cycling these two parts of the plan until you reach your goal weight and your jeans zip up effortlessly—it's that simple.

The Overnight Diet at a Glance

1-Day Power Up (Day 1)	Jump-starts weight loss overnight, accelerates fat burning, primes the body to respond optimally to the 6-Day Fuel Up.
6-Day Fuel Up (Days 2–7)	Keeps the fat coming off, feeds the muscles with the optimal amount of protein, fuels the body with an endless array of great-tasting, good-for-you foods for healthy weight loss without deprivation.

This combination primes the body, creating a sort of "metabolic marvel" that maximizes weight loss. So what happens inside the body when you alternate the 1-Day Power Up and the 6-Day Fuel Up?

Burn More Fat Faster

The Overnight Diet is formulated specifically to start incinerating fat faster than other diets. Most diets make you follow a lengthy initiation phase to stimulate weight loss. In today's "I want it now" society, who has time to wait around? This plan is engineered to turn on the process almost immediately. Thanks to the 1-Day Power Up, your body will begin using fat as energy as soon as 24 hours after you start the diet.

But in order to keep your body in fat-burning mode, you need to shift gears and follow the 6-Day Fuel Up. If you don't make the switch, the fat-burning process is more likely to stall. Years of testing on thousands of patients has shown that alternating back and forth between these two phases is the secret to keeping the fat coming off.

We need fat burning now more than ever. If you're reading this book, then you probably already know that America has a problem with fat—we've got too much of it. Nearly two-thirds of American adults are overweight and nearly one-third are obese. Middle-aged Americans are more likely to be obese than any other age group.

How much fat is too much? That's a question patients at the Nutrition and Weight Management Center at Boston Medical Center ask all the time. And it's understandable why. With so many millions of people expanding into the overweight and obese categories, it seems as if being overweight is the new normal. But as your parents probably told you when you were a teenager, "Just because everybody else is doing it doesn't mean you should."

One patient, Lydia, admitted that it took her a while to realize she had a weight problem because everybody in her family was overweight and many of her friends and neighbors were, too. Even though Lydia was more than 30 pounds above a healthy weight, she thought she was at a normal weight because that's what was normal in her social circle. But then she saw the Body Mass Index (BMI) chart. For decades, scientists have been using BMI as an indicator of a person's body fat and to determine if a person is underweight, normal weight, overweight, obese, or even morbidly obese. But because so many people think the same way Lydia did about being at a "normal" weight, it's better to think of it as a "healthy" weight. So forget normal, and get healthy.

With the BMI chart, it doesn't matter if you're the skinniest one

FIND YOUR BMI

Find your height in the left-hand column, then find your weight in the row to the right. Your BMI is at the top of that column.

BMI	Underweight	Healthy Weight						Overweight					Obese		Morbidly Obese
	<19	19	20	21	22	23	24	25	26	27	28	29	30	35	40
Height		Weight (in pounds)													
4'10"	<91	91	96	100	105	110	115	119	124	129	134	138	143	167	191
4'11"	<94	94	99	104	109	114	119	124	128	133	138	143	148	173	198
5'0"	<97	97	102	107	112	118	123	128	133	138	143	148	153	179	204
5'1"	<100	100	106	111	116	122	127	132	137	143	148	153	158	185	211
5'2"	<104	104	109	115	120	126	131	136	142	147	153	158	164	191	218
5'3"	<107	107	113	118	124	130	135	141	146	152	158	163	169	197	225
5'4"	<110	110	116	122	128	134	140	145	151	157	163	169	174	204	232
5'5"	<114	114	120	126	132	138	144	150	156	162	168	174	180	210	240
5'6"	<118	118	124	130	136	142	148	155	161	167	173	179	186	216	247
5'7"	<121	121	127	134	140	146	153	159	166	172	178	185	191	223	255
5'8"	<125	125	131	138	144	151	158	164	171	177	184	190	197	230	262
5'9"	<128	128	135	142	149	155	162	169	176	182	189	196	203	236	270
5'10"	<132	132	139	146	153	160	167	174	181	188	195	202	207	243	278
5'11"	<136	136	143	150	157	165	172	179	186	193	200	208	215	250	286
6'0"	<140	140	147	154	162	169	177	184	191	199	206	213	221	258	294
6'1"	<144	144	151	159	166	174	182	189	197	204	212	219	227	265	302
6'2"	<148	148	155	163	171	179	186	194	202	210	218	225	233	272	311
6'3"	<152	152	160	168	176	184	192	200	208	216	224	232	240	279	319
6'4"	<156	156	164	172	180	189	197	205	213	221	230	238	246	287	328

in a big family; it's all about the numbers. BMI is calculated using a ratio of height to weight. You can use "Find Your BMI," opposite, to see how your weight measures up. Do note, however, that BMI does have some limitations because it doesn't take into account a person's muscle mass. For example, an elite athlete who is very muscular and has low body fat may have a BMI that indicates overweight, when the athlete clearly does not need to lose weight. On the other end of the spectrum, someone with a very slight build, low muscle mass, and a spare tire may have a BMI that indicates healthy weight or even underweight, but he or she would benefit from losing fat and toning up.

Losing Weight by the Numbers

So what's your number? Whether your BMI is in the healthy range and you just want to maintain your weight or lose the last 5 pounds, you have 10 pounds to lose to get into the healthy range, or your BMI is over 30, this diet can work for you. About 450 patients come to the Nutrition and Weight Management Center each month, and they all have unique needs, just like you do. That's why this program has been created so it will work whether you want to lose a little or lose a lot. Just look at how it worked for Angie and her mom, Christina. Both wanted to lose weight, but each of them had very different goals.

Angie, twenty-eight, just wanted to drop about 10 pounds fast so she could fit into a form-fitting dress for her 10-year high school reunion, which was three weeks away. The dress had fit her perfectly when she bought it a couple months earlier, but after that, she had to travel to three week-long work conferences where fattening foods were served up buffet-style and the high-calorie cocktails were flowing. When she got back home and tried on her dress again, the zipper got stuck halfway up.

Christina, fifty-five, had been waging a war with fat for nearly thirty years and wanted to lose more than 40 pounds. She was very frustrated that she hadn't figured out a way to win the battle even though she felt like she'd been dieting her entire life.

They both started the very next day on the 1-Day Power Up and followed it up with the 6-Day Fuel Up. Overnight, Angie lost 1 pound and Christina dropped 2 pounds. By the end of the first week, Angie had lost 4 pounds and Christina was 6 pounds lighter. "We were both amazed how much our bodies had changed in just one week," Christina said. "That was just what I needed to keep going."

By the night of Angie's reunion, she had lost 11 pounds and 2 inches from her waist. "My dress zipped up so easily," she said. "It actually felt a little loose in the waist. I could have worn a smaller size!" Her mom, Christina, stuck with the program for six months and lost a total of 47 pounds, 5 inches off her midsection, and 7 inches off her hips. "I don't think my body has ever looked this good," she gushed at a follow-up appointment.

Get to Know Your Fat Cells

Many people think of the body's fat as the enemy, but your body needs fat cells to be healthy. Your body needs a place to store energy, and your fat cells do the job. Until recently, the theory was that we were all born with approximately the same number of fat cells—in the neighborhood of 10 billion—and that number would grow until we reached adulthood, at which time the number of fat cells would no longer budge. The belief was that if you consumed more calories than you expended, your fat cells would swell in size to accommodate that extra energy, but you wouldn't create any new fat cells. Based on this line of thinking, a lean person and someone who was 100 pounds overweight would have roughly the same number of fat cells, but the lean person's fat cells would be small and the overweight person's would be stretched like a balloon that's ready to pop. Now we know it isn't quite so simple.

New research is revealing that the secret life of fat cells is far more complex. Overeating does cause fat cells to swell up in size, but when stretched to the limit, some of them may divide and thus multiply, creating new fat cells. Theories now indicate that a lean adult might have about 10 to 20 billion fat cells, while an obese person might have as many as 100 billion. And then some people who cannot stretch their fat cells any further store fat in places such as the liver and muscle and develop diseases such as type 2 diabetes and cirrhosis of the liver.

Fat Burning 101

You know you want to burn fat, but how exactly does it happen? Getting that stubborn fat out of your body depends on a complicated bodily process, but to keep it simple, here are just the highlights. The same way your computer needs a power supply to keep it running, your body needs energy for daily life. It's what allows you to walk from the parking lot to your office at work, play with your toddler, or do housework. It's also required for a host of internal processes such as breathing, keeping your heart beating, and thinking. You may be surprised to discover that this last one is quite the calorie burner—when you're at rest, your brain consumes about 20 to 25 percent of your calories.

However, the body's number one source of energy for all these activities is glycogen, the form in which your body stores the carbohydrates you eat. The more daily activities performed, the more glycogen the body uses. If glycogen stores are completely depleted by these activities, then the body begins to burn fat as an alternate source of energy. When this happens, your body sends a signal to your fat cells to liberate their contents. The fat cells comply by releasing their "stuffing" in the form of free fatty acids that enter the bloodstream, something called *lipolysis*. The fatty acids are then shuttled to the muscles, internal organs, and other tissues, which burn them up for needed energy. This process is called *oxidation*. Once the fat is burned for energy, it's gone, and the fat cells that once housed it shrink. Skinnier fat cells translate into a skinnier you.

Turn Off Your "Fat Genes"

Did you know that your genetics may be working against you to make you fat? Genetic scientists have introduced the "Thrifty Gene Hypothesis," which suggests that in prehistoric times, certain genes helped our ancestors Caveman Joe and Cavewoman Jane thrive in times when food was scarce.

According to this theory, these genes played an important role in a natural cycle that alternated between feasting on food and then engaging in physical activity to hunt for their next meal. When Caveman Joe and Cavewoman Jane were successful at bringing home a wild animal for dinner, they would feast, and the so-called thrifty genes would go to work to store that food as fat. When the food supply ran out, Caveman Joe had to run, jump, and climb to hunt down their next meal while Cavewoman Jane walked, squatted down, and reached up high to gather plants and berries. That's when their fat stores would be burned as fuel. Feasting and storing fat; hunting and gathering for food and burning fat—that's the natural cycle our bodies were genetically programmed to follow and it's what kept Caveman Joe and Cavewoman Jane lean and athletic. (Have you ever seen a cave drawing of a fat caveman?)

Since those prehistoric times, our diets have changed dramatically. We now have an endless supply of food that we graze on constantly. And the only "hunting" required to acquire it is slowly strolling up and down the grocery store aisles. The nonstop eating and sedentary lifestyle mean that we no longer complete the natural eating cycle. Some scientists suggest that our diets have evolved, but our genetic programming hasn't caught up, and those genes that proved to be such a lifesaver for our ancestors are now making us fat and unhealthy. These experts contend that we've gotten stuck in feasting mode, and our genes are simply doing their job by storing more and more fat on our bodies. Not only is this expanding our waistlines, but it's also contributing to chronic diseases and poor health. Of course, in reality, it's far more complicated than this, but it is certainly possible that our genetics are working against us in the battle of the bulge.

Did you know...
Since the Industrial Revolution 200 years ago, countless fattening ingredients and foods have been introduced to our diets.

1798: Sucrose	1952: Frosted Flakes
1858: Feedlot-produced meats	1967: Big Mac
1886: Coca-Cola	1978: High-fructose corn syrup
About 1890: Refined grains	1978: Ben & Jerry's ice cream
1900: Hershey's bar	1985: Cinnabon
About 1900: Refined vegetable oils	1994: Wetzel's Pretzels
1918: Hydrogenated oils	2001: Deep-fried Snickers
1930: Toll-House cookies	About 2002: Fried Twinkies
1930: Twinkies	2009: Pizza Hut's Stuffed-Crust Pizza
1937: Krispy Kreme Doughnuts	2012: Jack in the Box's Bacon Shake
1941: M&M'S	

The Overnight Diet is the antidote for this problem. It signals your genes to take a break from their job of storing fat so your body can start burning it as fuel instead. Switching between the 1-Day Power Up and the 6-Day Fuel Up helps re-create the natural cycle our bodies were intended to follow so we can get our genes working *for* us rather than *against* us.

Put Your Fat Genes to Sleep

Have you ever blamed your genes for your weight troubles? You could be right, at least partly. To date, scientists have identified dozens of fat genes. In fact, they discovered 18 new ones in 2010 alone, and some say there could be as many as 100 of them. But we don't all possess all of them. The discovery of fat genes helps explain why weight problems tend to run in families. A review of 46 studies involving nearly 124,000 people combined showed that the more fat genes a person has, the more likely he or she is to be obese. People with over 38 fat genes weighed an average of 15 to 20 pounds more than those who had fewer than 22 fat genes.

Get the Skinny on Science

Were You Born This Way? Scientists are beginning to find the answers to this question, and more are on the way. In 2011, the National Institutes of Health gave a $2 million grant for a five-year study to investigate the impact of genetics on obesity and weight loss. Until the results of that study are revealed, here are some of the existing findings on what your parents might have had to do with your weight:

- Numerous studies on twins show that being obese is 40 to 75 percent hereditary.
- Researchers from London looked at 5,092 pairs of twins aged eight to eleven and found that their BMI and waist circumference were 77 percent hereditary.
- A study in the *Journal of Clinical Endocrinology & Metabolism* found that children born to a mother who had weight-loss surgery prior to pregnancy were less likely to be overweight than their siblings who were born before the mother had surgery. This suggests that a mother's weight during pregnancy may affect a developing fetus.

But this does not mean that just because your folks were fat you are doomed to be fat, too, or that there isn't anything you can do about it. Your genes are not your destiny! Your daily habits play a major role in what is called the "expression" of those genes. This means that your behaviors can effectively turn on or turn off those genes. Having doughnuts for breakfast and hitting the drive-thru for greasy fast-food lunches and dinners every day can power up those genes to start fulfilling their mission of making you fat. But give your body the delicious healthy foods you will be eating on this diet and it will help put those fat genes into the sleep mode.

Rev Up Metabolism

Metabolism is a complex bodily process that determines how quickly your body converts food into fuel and how fast it burns that fuel. It is part of the reason why some people can chow down at the all-you-can-eat buffet and still stay slim while the rest of us merely look on with envy. A sluggish metabolism is often blamed when diet after diet has failed.

Several factors play a role in determining the speed of your metabolism, including your age, gender, and genetics. After you hit age forty, your metabolism slows by about 5 percent each decade. Women tend to burn fewer calories than men because they typically have less muscle mass than men. And those genes you inherited from Mom and Dad also count. But so does your body composition and your activity level. One of the main reasons your metabolism slows is that, with age, people tend to lose muscle mass through a process called *sarcopenia*, but we'll get to that in Chapter 2.

Weight-loss physicians use a rather complicated equation to determine a person's resting basal metabolic rate (BMR). That's the number of calories your body uses just to perform all its basic functions, such as breathing, digesting, and keeping your blood circulating. There's no need to bore you with the math here, but basically it means that a woman who is 5-foot-5 and weighs 200 pounds burns more calories on those basic functions than a woman who is the same height but weighs only 125 pounds. Now let's say that 200-pound woman loses 50 pounds. This means her body now uses fewer calories on basic functions, so she needs to eat less to maintain her body weight.

When you carry extra weight, it causes your body to work harder to perform all the necessary processes of life. That's why, when you try a new diet that simply cuts calories, you probably lose weight easily at first, but then it gets harder and harder to keep it coming off. Your BMR naturally declines as you drop the weight. It simply doesn't have to work as hard to keep your body functioning. So even though you're consuming the same amount of calories on your diet, you may stop losing weight, which can make you want to quit dieting altogether.

Tales of the Measuring Tape

"I always thought it was my metabolism that was preventing me from losing weight. A couple of my girlfriends and I tried a few diets together and they all lost weight easily—of course they gained it all back!—but I would lose a few pounds then hit a plateau. I was ready to give up entirely and felt like I was destined to be fat for the rest of my life. Now I know why my metabolism was working against me. We were all eating the same number of calories per day, but because I weighed about 75 pounds less than they did to start, I dropped fewer pounds. Plus, even though I stuck within the calorie restrictions, I was eating foods and doing exercises that did nothing to boost metabolism. With the right foods and the easy workout on the Overnight Diet, I actually lost more weight than my girlfriends!"

—Andrea, 29, lost 28 pounds and four pants sizes

That's part of the reason there is no calorie counting on the Overnight Diet. The synergy of this combo diet is designed to avoid this common problem and *speed up* your metabolism as you lose weight so you can keep the pounds coming off—even if you've got age, gender, and genetics stacked against you. The nutritional makeup of the diet has been formulated with this specific goal in mind. You'll be eating lots of great-tasting, metabolism-boosting foods that will help you burn more calories faster. Plus, in Chapter 2, you will discover many more ways the Overnight Diet increases your metabolism.

MYTHBUSTERS

MYTH: Yo-yo dieting permanently slows your metabolism and makes it harder to burn calories. Many people think that because they have repeatedly lost weight through dieting and then gained it all back, their metabolism is ruined and will forever after be stuck in low gear. While it is true that some diets may temporarily wreak havoc with your metabolism, their effects don't last.

Several studies have been published that put this myth to rest. In one, Canadian researchers looked at fifty-two overweight women who had been yo-yo dieters for an average of 18 years. They calculated the women's resting metabolic rate then compared that number with what their resting metabolic rate would normally be based on their ages, heights, and weights. In more than 92 percent of the women, there was no difference.

This doesn't mean that weight cycling, as doctors refer to yo-yo dieting, is okay or healthy. In fact, it can have detrimental effects on your health. But the takeaway message here is that even if you have been a lifelong yo-yo dieter, you can still whip your metabolism back into shape by following the Overnight Diet.

Reduce Bloating by Enhancing Insulin Sensitivity

Did you know that having high levels of the hormone insulin can cause the body to retain extra water, which can make you feel bloated? The Overnight Diet is engineered to produce a dramatic reduction in the body's production of insulin. Lowering insulin levels flushes excess water out of the body to help get rid of that puffiness. Without that extra water weight, your body will become more defined as you lose weight. Who knows, you just might have a six-pack lying underneath that bloat.

You may be wondering if losing water weight is good for your health. The answer is yes, as long as you're flushing out *excess* water. We all need to be properly hydrated for optimal health, and this diet will provide you with adequate fluids. It's the excess fluid retention that gives you that bloated look and that stresses your body and health. Too much fluid in your system strains your body's vital organs by making them work harder. When you release those extra stores of water, your body works more efficiently and you shrink down in size more easily.

MYTHBUSTERS
MYTH: When you lose water weight, you will regain it quickly. This myth may be true with other diets on which you lose water weight during an initiation phase, only to regain it because the post-initiation foods you're eating don't reduce insulin levels. The 1-Day Power Up sparks that initial water weight loss, and the 6-Day Fuel Up keeps the weight from coming back. Alternating back and forth between these two parts of the Overnight Diet enhances something called insulin sensitivity. This means that insulin is working effectively at its primary job of regulating blood sugar, which helps keep water from accumulating in your body to prevent unwanted bloating. The 1-Day Power Up dramatically reduces insulin production, which enhances insulin sensitivity, and the 6-Day Fuel Up maintains insulin sensitivity at a high level to keep you from regaining water weight.

Boost Human Growth Hormone, Your Body's Natural Flab Fighter

Human growth hormone (HGH) is one of the most important natural hormones in the human body. Produced by the pituitary gland in the brain, it is involved in a variety of essential bodily functions, including reducing body fat, protecting lean muscle mass, and maintaining metabolic balance. The higher the levels of HGH, the better the body performs these duties. With age, levels of growth hormone dramatically decline and have been associated with weight gain, muscle loss, wrinkles, weakness, and more. If you've watched the news or read the sports page recently, you're probably familiar with HGH. Athletes, celebrities, and people looking for the fountain of youth are reportedly taking it for performance enhancement, injury recovery, weight loss, and anti-aging. And supplement manufacturers are trying to cash in with products promising to stimulate HGH production.

Let's be perfectly clear here: The Overnight Diet does not suggest that you take HGH supplements to help you achieve your weight-loss goals.

But the Overnight Diet will help boost HGH levels naturally. This diet, and the 1-Day Power Up in particular, has been engineered to kick HGH into high gear so you can get slimmer faster. Researchers at the Intermountain Medical Center for Heart Health in Utah presented findings at the 2011 annual scientific sessions of the American College of Cardiology confirming earlier evidence showing that following a diet similar to the 1-Day Power Up for just 24 hours significantly accelerates production of HGH. How much? In women HGH levels jumped by an average of 1,300 percent, and in men levels skyrocketed nearly 2,000 percent. This doesn't mean that this diet is going to make you look twenty years younger overnight, but follow it to the letter and you will be leaner, feel more vibrant, *and* look more youthful.

MYTHBUSTERS

MYTH: If I want to get thin fast, I can just get liposuction and keep eating whatever I want. Sorry, folks, but liposuction is not the answer. Yes, liposuction can produce a rapid change in appearance—although the procedure is associated with significant swelling that can take six weeks or more to completely subside. But it is not the answer for long-term weight loss. Liposuction doesn't prime your body for fat burning, doesn't flip the switch to rev your metabolism to keep weight from coming back, and doesn't boost levels of HGH to fight flab. And according to research in the *New England Journal of Medicine*, liposuction doesn't decrease your body's production of insulin to prevent bloat and doesn't reduce your risk factors for heart disease or type 2 diabetes. Liposuction certainly doesn't teach you how to eat to keep fat off for the rest of your life, and it costs about $3,000 per area.

Prevent Plateaus

Plateaus are one of the most common roadblocks to weight-loss success. For some people, it's their metabolism slowing down that causes the scale to get stuck. For others, it's sheer boredom eating the same few foods from a diet's "approved" list that causes progress to stall. Whatever your reasons may be for hitting plateaus, this diet will make them a thing of the past. On the Overnight Diet, every 7 days you can lose up to 2 pounds overnight with the 1-Day Power Up to shake up those plateaus week in and week out. Plateau problem solved!

Maria, thirty-one, had tried diet after diet but could never lose those last 5 pounds to get to her goal weight. "I thought I was going to be stuck with those stubborn pounds forever," she said. But switching from the 1-Day Power Up to the 6-Day Fuel Up did the trick. "It worked," she said. "Finally reaching my goal weight after all this time feels so incredible. I look better than ever, and I feel better than ever, too."

Stave Off Hunger Pangs

Is it really possible to lose weight and not feel hungry while doing it? You bet! The Overnight Diet is specifically formulated to give you the results you want without the deprivation. This aspect is critical because feeling deprived while dieting increases cravings and bingeing, which can sabotage weight-loss efforts. Thinking that you can never indulge in the foods you love most can also be downright depressing and demotivating. This plan was formulated with these issues in mind, which is why you won't go hungry, and you won't have to give up your favorite foods, such as bread, spaghetti, and burgers.

The Overnight Diet emphasizes nutrition that is high in lean protein and fiber, both of which have been shown to increase satiety. That means they help keep you feeling full longer, so your stomach doesn't start to rumble soon after meals. Plus, you'll have an all-you-can-eat option for fruits and nonstarchy vegetables. There are no limits on these good-for-you foods so you never have to go hungry while dropping pounds.

Get the Skinny on the Science

Satiety and the Fullness Factor How do we know which foods provide the greatest level of satiety? One of the most interesting studies on foods and fullness comes from Suzanna Holt and fellow researchers at the University of Sydney. In an experiment, Holt and her team fed human test subjects a variety of foods to determine which types of food made them feel fullest the longest. According to their findings, foods with high amounts of fiber, protein, and/or water tend to be the most satisfying and are the best at preventing hunger. By contrast, foods that contain high amounts of sugar, fat, and/or starch tend to provide less satiety and may lead to hunger pangs soon after eating.

Eat More Foods, Lose More Weight

Most diets start with initiation phases that severely restrict what foods can be eaten; some turn antioxidant-rich fruit into a forbidden food, while others allow for little more than protein at first. But it's nearly impossible to stick with these types of diets. That's why this plan lets you enjoy so many of the foods you love right from the start. You won't have to cut out all carbs, forgo dairy, or slice fruit from your diet.

What will you be eating on the Overnight Diet? During the 1-Day Power Up, you'll be enjoying a unique blend of tasty, filling foods that you'll find in Chapter 3, and you'll learn all about the great foods you'll be eating on the 6-Day Fuel Up in Chapter 4. But just know this for now: From the get-go, you'll be eating lean protein, low-fat dairy, healthy fats, and "lean carbs"—whole grains, and all-you-can-eat fruits and nonstarchy vegetables. And there's also room in this diet for the things you really love, including dessert and wine.

The guidelines for eating are so simple with the Overnight Diet, you can forget about any arbitrary restrictions. Some diets tell you that the secret to weight loss is to stop eating carbs after a certain time of day, but there is no scientific basis for these claims! Rest assured, your body is just as capable of metabolizing the calories from a slice of whole-grain bread or an orange at 8 p.m. as it is at 11 a.m.

Some diets claim that there are super-weight-loss powers in specific foods and encourage you to focus on those particular foods every single day, but these are just gimmicks. Scientific research shows us that there are hundreds of wonderful foods that can help you trim down, and you will find all those foods in this book. Why force you to eat only a few of them? This diet gives you free rein to find the fat-busting, metabolism-boosting foods that you love. After all, you're more likely to stick with a plan that lets you eat the foods you enjoy than one that makes you eat the same thing day in and day out. With dishes such as Beefy Mushroom Burgers, Rosemary Pork Roast, Italian "Sausage" Pizza, Diana's Magnificent Hearty Pancakes, and yummy desserts such as Apple Cranberry Crisp and Lemon Cheesecake Parfait, eating healthy is a pleasure.

Get the Skinny on the Science

Say Hello to Lean Carbs Carbohydrates have gotten a bad rap in recent years, but the research shows that the low-carb craze got it wrong. Carbs are essential to a healthy diet and to losing weight and keeping it off. The Overnight Diet emphasizes "lean carbs." These are whole grains, fruits, and nonstarchy vegetables, and they are a key component of this get-slim plan. A 2009 study in the *Journal of the American Dietetic Association* evaluated the diets of 4,451 adults and found that those consuming the most lean carbs were the least likely to be overweight or obese and those who ate the fewest lean carbs were the heaviest.

Enhance Motivation

Nicole, forty-four, couldn't lose the 35 pounds she'd gained since having her second child almost ten years earlier. She'd tried to diet and would lose some weight in the first few weeks, but then her motivation would wane and she'd give up. Nicole isn't alone. Nearly every patient at the Nutrition and Weight Management Center at Boston Medical Center has struggled with staying motivated while trying to lose weight. Most of them say that their enthusiasm starts to slip away when they hit one of those pesky plateaus or, even worse, gain a few pounds while dieting. And who can blame them? When the scale doesn't cooperate, you can feel as if all your efforts are in vain.

With this diet, the pounds will keep coming off each week, so it's easy to stay motivated. Just ask Nicole. After losing 38 pounds—3 more pounds than her goal weight!—on the Overnight Diet, she said, "Because I kept losing weight each week, it kept me motivated to keep going. That's never happened to me before."

Success is a powerful motivator. And you'll likely get a jolt of it after just one day. When you wake up the morning after doing the 1-Day Power Up and are already lighter, it makes you want to keep going. And when you see more weight come off with the 6-Day Fuel Up, it only adds to your confidence. Then you start over again with the 1-Day Power Up, when you can lose up to another 2 pounds. Having that powerful day in the plan is so important in keeping your motivation humming.

Achieve Lifetime Weight Control

The Overnight Diet's combination of these two scientifically proven weight-loss methods will help you keep your weight under control *for the rest of your life!* This isn't a restrictive plan; the Overnight Diet is a way of life. The basic concept of alternating from the 1-Day Power Up to the 6-Day Fuel Up is something you can easily do for years to come and is the answer to keeping weight off for good.

Charlene, fifty-one, who lost over 40 pounds as a patient, has been doing it for four years now, and she says it's become second nature to her. "I can't imagine eating any other way now," she said. "After reaching my goal weight, I made a few tweaks, but still follow the 1-Day/6-Day cycle. And now my husband does it, too, even though he doesn't need to lose weight. We just love the way everything tastes and like the way it makes us feel."

Like Charlene, once you reach your goal weight, you, too, can make a few simple adjustments to the Overnight Diet to make it a plan for the rest of your life. (Check out Chapter 11 for details.)

CHAPTER 2

Adding More Muscle to the Overnight Diet

Taking two proven weight-loss methods—a temporary break from solid food and the Protein Sparing Modified Fast—reengineering them, and combining them into one plan are only part of how this diet will turn your body into a powerful fat burner. There is another component that takes the synergy of this hybrid diet and makes it even more powerful: preserving lean muscle.

The amount of lean muscle in your body is one of the key elements in setting your body's metabolic rate and determining how quickly you use calories. The more lean muscle you have, the better your body is at burning fuel. The less you have, the slower your metabolism. The problem is our diets and lifestyles are robbing our bodies of the muscle that we need to help us incinerate fat and slim down.

Remember the Shrinking Muscle Syndrome we discussed in the Introduction? It's the loss of lean muscle that occurs naturally as you get older. Starting at age thirty, muscle mass begins to decrease by about 1 percent each year. But it is also an unwelcome side effect of losing weight on many popular diets. On low-carb diets, you will lose some fat, but you will also lose some muscle mass. And those old-fashioned low-fat diets that are high in carbohydrates and low in protein? They can also rob the body of lean muscle.

The Shrinking Muscle Syndrome is the giant pothole that sends you veering off the path to fast results and permanent weight loss, and derails your efforts for a slimmer, trimmer, healthier you. Let's explore how it causes fat burning to sputter.

The Shrinking Muscle Syndrome

When the Shrinking Muscle Syndrome occurs, you may not even know it at first. But after some time, you may start to notice that walking seems to take a lot more effort than it used to. Climbing stairs may leave you huffing and puffing. You may even begin to feel that it's a bit trickier to maintain your balance. But before you ever notice these telltale external signs, a whole barrage of changes have already started taking place inside your body—changes that rob your body of muscle tissue and sabotage your ability to lose weight and burn fat.

Tales of the Measuring Tape

"I could barely get up the stairs to my bedroom without gasping for air, and I felt like I was dragging all the time. I thought that it was just because of all the extra weight I was carrying around. I had no idea that it was also due to the fact that my muscles were disappearing. When I learned about the Shrinking Muscle Syndrome, it really made sense. Gaining muscle is what helped me lose the weight and get into the best shape of my life. Now I can run up the stairs!"

—Madison, 39, lost 92 pounds

To help you understand the chaos that occurs inside your body, let's look at the major players on your muscle-building team and the changes that keep them from doing their job.

• **Mitochondria.** Inside your body's cells are mitochondria—tiny engines that take in nutrients and use them to provide energy. All of your cells have some mitochondria, but your muscles are absolutely packed with them, which gives your muscles the energy to walk, run, jump, push, pull, lift, and so on. Your body is constantly regenerating mitochondria so it can create the energy your muscles need to perform. But as you age, this process slows down and two things happen: Your body regenerates fewer mitochondria, and the mitochondria you do have get a bit sluggish. When your mitochondria no longer perform their job of converting nutrients into usable energy as efficiently as they used to, it results in less muscle tissue and slower response times from your muscles.

• **HGH.** In Chapter 1, you saw how HGH helps fight flab naturally. HGH plays an essential role in cell development and regeneration, both of which are important for preserving lean muscle mass, as you will learn later in this chapter. Higher levels of HGH have been associated with increases in lean muscle mass and reductions in body fat. As you age, the body's production of HGH slows to a crawl, and your muscles begin to shrink and weaken.

• **Insulin-like growth factor-1 (IGF-1).** IGF-1, a natural hormone produced in the liver, promotes cell growth and regeneration, particularly cells within the muscles. When levels of HGH rise, the liver pumps out more IGF-1, which has been associated with increases in lean muscle mass and decreases in body fat. Adequate levels of IGF-1 have been found to help in the prevention of the age-related degeneration of muscles.

When IGF-1 levels are insufficient, however, muscles tend to wither away and body fat increases. Low levels of IGF-1 can be due to many factors, including nutritional deficiencies, such as those caused by extreme calorie cutting.

In essence, the Shrinking Muscle Syndrome decreases your body's ability to perform muscle repair and to generate muscle tissue. It reduces the concentration of your body's natural fat-burning hormones, including HGH and IGF-1. Not only does your body generate less of these hormones, but it also responds more weakly to the hormones that are already circulating in the body.

Fat invades your muscles. Most people think that as we gain weight, the fat basically sits on top of our muscles, creating unsightly lumps and bulges under the skin. But we now know that isn't entirely true. New imaging studies reveal that as your BMI rises, fat infiltrates your muscles, further decreasing their ability to perform the most basic functions. Take a look at Figures 2.1 and 2.2 to see just how much fat invades the muscles as BMI increases. In these images, the dark areas are muscle, and the light areas are fat.

Fat Within Muscle Fiber at Different BMIs

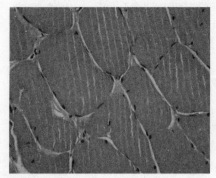 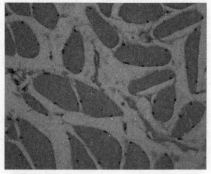

FIG.2.1 *BMI 19*   FIG.2.2 *BMI 35*

(Photos courtesy of Tom Storer, PhD, Boston University School of Medicine)

Once your body starts losing lean muscle mass and experiencing a decrease in the quality of the muscle fiber, it puts you on the expressway to Blubberville. Weakened, withered muscles impair your ability to function, which makes you more likely to join the growing ranks of couch potatoes, which in turn makes your muscles even weaker. It's another one of those vicious cycles that sabotage weight loss. What makes it even worse is if you continue to eat the way you always have while these changes are taking place in your muscles, the pounds start to accumulate quickly.

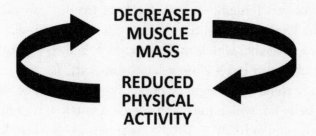

DECREASED MUSCLE MASS

REDUCED PHYSICAL ACTIVITY

Unfortunately, with the Shrinking Muscle Syndrome, packing on the pounds is only the tip of the iceberg. Muscle loss can lead to a host of other metabolic problems that make losing weight nearly impossible. If the Overnight Diet works synergistically to create a sort of "metabolic marvel" that helps you burn fat and lose weight, the Shrinking Muscle Syndrome does just the opposite. It creates a metabolic *mess* that causes fat to stick stubbornly to your body.

In particular, the Shrinking Muscle Syndrome is associated with insulin resistance, the metabolic syndrome, and inflammation—all conditions that detract from your body's ability to burn fat. Many of the patients at the Nutrition and Weight Management Center at Boston Medical Center have one or more of these problems, and what's really scary is that the vast majority of them don't even know it! It's like they have been waging a war against fat for years and years without realizing that these chronic conditions are fighting against them. No wonder they have such a tough time losing weight.

Here's a quick look at how these conditions associated with the Shrinking Muscle Syndrome sabotage weight loss.

Insulin resistance. Insulin resistance is a condition in which your body produces the hormone insulin but doesn't use it efficiently. Insulin, which is produced by the pancreas, helps your body's cells use glucose for energy. Let's say you eat a burger, fries, and a shake at your favorite fast-food spot. Your body converts that food into glucose, and your pancreas starts pumping out insulin so you can use that glucose as energy.

But with insulin resistance, your body doesn't use the hormone efficiently, so your pancreas keeps spewing out more and more insulin. As you remember, high levels of insulin can cause water retention. That's why insulin resistance is associated with carrying extra water weight, which makes you look and feel bloated. Insulin resistance also has a close relationship with fat and makes you more likely to be overweight or obese. It is linked especially closely to extra belly fat, which means that even if you lose weight on some other diets, you're likely to still be stuck with those love handles or muffin top. Insulin resistance can also lead to excess amounts of glucose in the bloodstream and can set the stage for prediabetes or type 2 diabetes.

Tales of the Measuring Tape

"I didn't have a lot of weight to lose, but whenever I cut calories and lost a few pounds, I still felt bloated and could never get rid of that jiggly belly that would spill over the top of my jeans. I was shocked when my blood tests revealed that I had insulin resistance and was prediabetic! That was a big part of the problem and no amount of simple calorie cutting was going to fix that."

—Sophie, 33, lost 12 pounds and 2 inches off her waist

So what does the Shrinking Muscle Syndrome have to do with insulin resistance? Your muscles play a starring role in your body's ability to use insulin. The more lean muscle you have, the more effectively your body uses insulin. The muscle loss that occurs with age or from trying to lose weight with many popular diets reduces your body's ability to use insulin. The end result? More bloating, stubborn fat, and possibly type 2 diabetes.

And once again, it's a double-edged sword. Muscle loss contributes to insulin resistance, and insulin resistance also promotes muscle wasting. It's like driving onto one of those circular roundabouts and then picking up so much speed that you can't safely navigate to any of the exits. You get stuck going around and around and around. And once you get trapped in that loop, it's a speedy trip to another spare tire around your midsection.

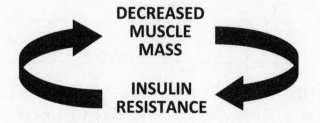

Get the Skinny on the Science

The Shrinking Muscle Syndrome–Insulin Resistance Loop In a 2010 issue of *PloS ONE*, a team of scientists from UCLA analyzed data from 14,528 people to see if muscle loss plays a role in insulin resistance. They found that muscle wasting was associated with insulin resistance not only in obese people but also in people who were not seriously overweight. This means that even if you are losing weight on a diet, you could be setting the stage for insulin resistance if you are also losing lean muscle on that diet. And that will make it much harder for you to keep that weight off.

Metabolic syndrome. Metabolic syndrome is a cluster of conditions that increase your risk for heart disease, stroke, and diabetes. The conditions associated with metabolic syndrome include the following:

High waist measurement. Having too much blubber on your belly, or having an "apple" shape, is a greater health risk than if you have a "pear" shape. The following waist measurements are associated with metabolic syndrome:

Waist Size

Women	35" or higher
Men	40" or higher

High triglycerides. Triglycerides are a type of fat in the blood. Having high levels of this type of fat increases your risk for the syndrome.

Triglycerides

Optimal	150 or less
High	150 or higher

Low HDL cholesterol. HDL is often referred to as the "good" cholesterol. Its primary job is to sweep cholesterol out of your arteries so blood can flow freely. When HDL levels are low, there is a greater chance of cholesterol building up in the arteries and potentially creating a blockage or causing heart disease.

HDL Levels

	Women	*Men*
Optimal	60 and above	60 and above
Low	Less than 50	Less than 40

High fasting blood sugar. Having a high fasting blood sugar level is an indicator of prediabetes or diabetes and is associated with increased risk for serious disease.

Fasting Blood Sugar

Optimal	Below 100
High	100 or higher

High blood pressure. Your blood pressure measures the force of the blood as it pumps through your arteries. High blood pressure means your body is pumping blood with greater force. This condition is associated with a higher likelihood for heart disease and stroke.

Blood Pressure

Optimal	Below 120/80
High	130/85 or higher

Having any one of these conditions alone puts you at increased risk for disease, but doesn't mean you have metabolic syndrome.

Having *all* these conditions together is what really ratchets up the health risk and makes it almost impossible for you to lose weight and keep it off.

Being overweight, and in particular having a large belly, has long been associated with the metabolic syndrome, but guess what? Scientists have found that low muscle mass and decreased strength are also important risk factors for metabolic syndrome. This means that the Shrinking Muscle Syndrome can put you on the road to this dangerous condition. So can losing weight—and muscle—on some other diets.

Inflammation. Inflammation is the body's natural response when we are exposed to foreign invaders, such as a splinter, a virus, bacteria, or toxins. We need it on a short-term basis to fight disease and infection. But inflammation can become chronic, which has been associated with heart disease, obesity, diabetes, Alzheimer's disease, and more.

Scientists are just beginning to understand the link between fat, inflammation, and muscle wasting. For example, scientific evidence suggests that fat tissue, especially abdominal fat, produces chemicals that promote inflammation. And emerging research is finding that chronic inflammation also accelerates muscle wasting. For example, in the *Journal of Applied Physiology*, a study from Italian researchers examined the link between obesity, muscle strength, and inflammation in 378 men and 493 women. The scientists looked at their waist measurements, tested their strength using a handgrip device, and checked their blood levels for inflammation markers. The results showed that the people with higher waist measurements and lower strength also had higher levels of inflammation. The researchers concluded that abdominal fat directly affects inflammation, which in turn negatively affects muscle strength.

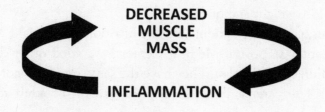

DECREASED MUSCLE MASS

INFLAMMATION

Common Causes of the Shrinking Muscle Syndrome

What shifts your body into the Shrinking Muscle Syndrome gear? Of course, age has a hand in muscle wasting, but that's not all. Your diet could be putting you in danger of this condition. It may surprise you that a low-carb diet could pose a problem with muscle loss, but I'll tell you how it could happen. In addition, a lack of physical activity, and in particular a lack of strength training, can rob your body of muscle tissue.

The Diet–Shrinking Muscle Syndrome Connection

If you're like most people who are trying to lose weight, you may think you're doing your body a favor by following a typical low-calorie, low-fat, or low-carb diet. But some of the most popular diet plans will ultimately fail to give you the sleek body you want and will leave your body feeling flabby instead of fit. Research from my mentors Dr. Blackburn and Dr. Bistrian found that low protein consumption is also associated with muscle loss.

Many low-fat diets are also low in protein and high in carbohydrates. Many low-calorie diets offer no recommendations on daily protein intake, so you may not be getting enough of it to stave off muscle loss. And those low-carb diets? If you're cutting out healthful, whole-grain carbs while eating limitless amounts of fat and not consciously eating an adequate amount of protein, it could take a toll on your muscle mass. Not eating enough protein can derail your dieting efforts because it sets the stage for the Shrinking Muscle Syndrome and all the problems that come with it that make it so hard to lose weight and burn fat.

Thousands of the patients at the Nutrition and Weight Management Center at Boston Medical Center have tried other diets but still couldn't lose the flab. They have the same problem: not enough protein! They aren't alone. Nearly 40 percent of adult men and women eat less protein than the current Recommended Dietary Allowance (RDA) of a minimum of 0.8 grams per kilogram of ideal body weight per day. And the Overnight Diet recommends more, as you will see below.

Tales of the Measuring Tape

"I was on one of those low-fat, low-protein, high-carb diets and couldn't figure out why I wasn't reaching my goal weight. I was doing everything it said to do. When I told Dr. Apovian what I was eating, she informed me that I wasn't getting enough protein. When I started eating the right amount of protein, I started losing weight fast... and I didn't feel starving anymore!"

—Randi, 27, lost 14 pounds

So what does protein intake have to do with maintaining lean muscle mass? A lot! Protein is the building block for your body's muscles. And every day of your life your muscles are going through a never-ending cycle of breaking down the proteins within and regenerating new proteins to replace them. To create these new proteins, your muscles need amino acids. Your body makes some of these amino acids on its own, but nine of them can be derived only from the foods you eat. These nine are called "essential amino acids."

Animal protein (meat, poultry, fish, seafood, eggs, and milk) and soy foods contain all nine of the essential amino acids that your muscles need for rebuilding. When you don't eat enough protein, your body doesn't get the amino acids it needs to regenerate new proteins, and it will continue breaking down your muscle, which ultimately leads to muscle wasting. Unlike carbohydrates and fat, the human body does not store amino acids for later use. This means that amino acids—in the form of protein—must be consumed *every day* in order to maintain muscle mass. Even one day of eating inadequate amounts of protein kick-starts the muscle-wasting process.

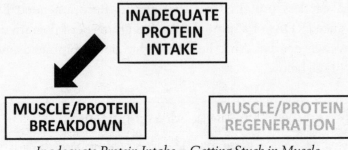

Inadequate Protein Intake = Getting Stuck in Muscle
Breakdown Mode

What's Exercise Got to Do with the Shrinking Muscle Syndrome?

Remember the Thrifty Gene Hypothesis? It is the theory that your genetic programming says your body is designed to follow a pattern of feasting on food and then hunting and gathering for your next meal. The 1-Day Power Up and 6-Day Fuel Up have been engineered to help re-create that natural cycle, but there's one more piece that fits into that cycle: physical activity. After all, when you have to hunt for your food, you have to run, jump, and maybe even climb a tree. And gathering requires you to walk, bend, squat, and stretch. And then if you're successful, you have to haul your dinner back home. That's a lot of work!

Here's how hunting and gathering work in today's society: Some of us sit on the couch and use our cell phone or computer to order takeout. Twenty minutes later, the doorbell rings, and we get off the couch to answer the door, then "haul" the food back to the couch to eat it. Successful hunt and gather! Some of us grab our keys, drive to the nearest fast-food joint, order from the drive-thru, and eat right there in our cars. Successful hunt and gather! Some of us drive to the grocery store, shuffle up and down the aisles, fill our carts with our favorite foods, then drive back home, pop something in the microwave, and chow down. Successful hunt and gather!

Aside from it being a piece of cake to hunt down food in the modern world, it's the kinds of foods we're hunting and gathering that are making it harder to stop eating. We tend to gather and eat too much sugar and fat, which seems to produce inflammation throughout the body and even in the brain. In particular, inflammation seems to affect a region of the brain called the hypothalamus, which is your appetite and satiety center. With inflammation here, your satiety mechanism goes haywire and stops sending you the signals that tell you you're full, so you keep eating, and eating, and eating.

Hunting and gathering in today's world is akin to shooting fish in a barrel. It's far too easy and requires barely any physical effort. The same effect can be seen in the rest of the tasks in our daily lives. Our society's focus on convenience has effectively turned us into sedentary beings: Less than one-third of U.S. adults engage in regular leisure-time physical activity, and 10 percent of U.S. adults do no physical activity at all in their leisure time, and that's stripping our bodies of muscle. Scientists have shown that a sedentary lifestyle accelerates muscle wasting.

But being inactive isn't the only way to make your muscles wither away. Did you know that the exercise recommendations of many popular diets could actually be preventing you from reaching your weight-loss goals? And even worse, could be putting you in danger of muscle wasting? For decades, diets have been promoting aerobic exercise as the best way to burn calories and shed pounds. But the combination of very low-calorie diets with hours of cardio may be a recipe for the Shrinking Muscle Syndrome because it can put the body into a catabolic state in which it robs the muscles for fuel. During aerobic exercise, muscle proteins are broken down for energy. Adequate nutrition, and in particular protein, is necessary to regenerate those muscle proteins. If you don't consume adequate amounts of nutrients, especially protein, then the muscles will begin to wither.

The Overnight Diet: The Shrinking Muscle Syndrome Solution

The Overnight Diet has been designed specifically to preserve lean muscle mass so you can avoid the Shrinking Muscle Syndrome and finally reach your weight-loss goals. It starts with getting adequate protein. Well, what's adequate?

The current RDA for protein is 0.8 grams per kilogram of body weight per day. But that's not enough. Based on the research of Dr. George Blackburn and Dr. Bruce Bistrian, pioneers in the field of nutrition and metabolism, as well as my own research and experience with thousands of weight-loss patients, this amount is too low to optimize weight loss or muscle up metabolism. To fuel fat burning, the Overnight Diet draws from the proven high-protein concept that was first advocated by the Blackburn-Bistrian team and that has been retooled to provide results for the community-dwelling individual. Very simply, you need to almost double the RDA's recommendations and consume a *minimum* of 1.5 grams of protein per kilogram of ideal body weight. This is called your Daily Protein Requirement or DPR as we will refer to it, and it's a critical component of this diet.

Let's say your ideal body weight is 130 pounds, which equals 59 kilograms. At that weight, the RDA indicates you should be eating approximately 47 grams of protein per day, or about 7 ounces (7 grams of protein equals 1 ounce of protein). But experience and research show that this isn't enough to prevent muscle loss. On the Overnight Diet, you would be eating a *minimum* of about 89 grams, or about 13 ounces, of protein per day. What does that look like on your plate? You'll get the specifics in the coming chapters, but just to give you an idea for now: a breakfast that includes an egg and spinach omelet with fat-free cheddar cheese; a 5-ounce grilled chicken breast wrap for lunch; and a 5-ounce broiled salmon filet for dinner would fill your protein needs. Of course, you would be rounding out those meals with other healthy foods.

Knowing your individual DPR is essential for success on this program. You can use "Find Your DPR" in Chapter 4, pages 68–69, to help you determine yours.

With an adequate amount of protein in your diet, your body will replenish the amino acids needed to halt the breakdown of your muscles and rebuild them. And by harnessing the power of protein to preserve lean muscle mass, you will be pushing fat burning into overdrive.

Get the Skinny on the Science

The Power of Protein In a seminal scientific paper published in the *Journal of the American Medical Association* in 1978, Dr. Blackburn described the safety and efficacy of a protein-sparing modified fast—a low-calorie diet that included 1.5 grams of protein per kilogram of ideal body weight per day.

In a follow-up study published in the *Journal of Clinical Investigation* in 1984, Dr. Blackburn, Dr. Bistrian, and colleagues compared the effects of a very low-calorie diet on nitrogen balance with either 0.8 or 1.5 grams of protein per kilogram of ideal body weight per day. Eating 0.8 grams of protein per kilogram of ideal body weight per day disrupted the dieters' nitrogen balance, but consuming 1.5 grams of protein per kilogram of ideal body weight per day resulted in optimal nitrogen balance. Nitrogen is a compound that is used to measure a person's level of amino acids. When nitrogen balance is optimal, it means that a person has an adequate level of amino acids in the body for proper muscle regeneration. When nitrogen balance is skewed, it typically means there are not enough amino acids in the body to halt muscle breakdown.

Research on protein consumption and the maintenance of lean muscle has continued since Dr. Blackburn's first paper on the topic. A 2011 study from the University of Illinois shows that eating protein throughout the day is key to losing weight without sacrificing muscle. The study followed the dieting efforts of 31 postmenopausal women, all of whom ate a 1,400-calorie diet for six months. The women were divided into two groups, one of which received a powdered whey protein supplement twice a day and one that received a placebo containing an equal number of calories in carbohydrates. By the end of the study, the women who had consumed the additional protein had lost 3.9 percent more weight and had a relative gain of 5.8 percent more thigh muscle volume than women who didn't eat as much protein.

Pump Up Your Muscles to Power Up Fat Burning

Because maintaining and adding lean muscle mass is the key to rapid weight loss that lasts, you won't have to dedicate big chunks of your day to aerobics in order to burn fat on this plan. Instead, you will be focusing on getting lean muscles through strength training. But don't worry. This is no run-of-the-mill weight-lifting routine. The same way this plan combines two diets into one for maximum results, it also integrates two exercise concepts into one to create a dynamic fat-burning session that lets you quickly strengthen and resculpt your body without ever having to lift a barbell or spend hours on the treadmill.

Tales of the Measuring Tape

"You mean I can develop lean muscles and burn more fat without going to the gym or lifting heavy weights? Thank you!"
—Amanda, 44, lost 19 pounds

This unique workout plan relies on a growing body of research showing that combining resistance training with short cardio bursts, called "Rev Up Blasts" here, into one workout burns far more body fat compared to doing strength training and cardio separately. For example, a pair of recent studies in the *Journal of Strength and Conditioning Research* compared the fat-burning effects of two types of workout routines. The first was a standard routine, including a weight-training session followed by an aerobic workout. The second was an integrated workout, in which people alternated weight-training exercises with high-intensity sprints. The combo workout outpaced the traditional routine in every area, including endurance, muscle strength, and flexibility. But most excitingly, the people who did the hybrid workout lost almost ten times more body fat compared to those who did the traditional workout.

The fun, fast-paced Quickie Rev Up takes only 21 minutes four times a week, requires no equipment, and can be tailored for all fitness levels, whether you're a workout newbie or a longtime exerciser. The easy-to-follow moves strengthen nearly every major muscle group in the body while improving balance and flexibility at the same time. And they are designed to help you move better so you can do all the things you want to do, like spring up off the floor after playing with your toddler, take your dog for a brisk walk, or go dancing with your spouse. It's fun, it's fast, and it's functional for everyday life.

Building lean muscle with this strength-training program will fuel fat burning by boosting your metabolism and by helping you avoid the conditions that keep you fat, including insulin resistance and the metabolic syndrome. You have seen how the Shrinking Muscle Syndrome increases your risk for these conditions. New research is showing that when you add lean muscle to your body, you can prevent or even reverse them.

Several studies have shown that having low muscle mass is a risk factor for insulin resistance. But until 2011, no scientific research had attempted to find out if increasing muscle mass could reduce that risk. That's when a pair of researchers from UCLA analyzed data from 13,644 people to test this concept. In their study, which appeared in a 2011 issue of the *Journal of Clinical Endocrinology & Metabolism*, they found that for every 10 percent increase in muscle mass there was an 11 percent reduction in the incidence of insulin resistance.

In the journal *Metabolism*, Australian researchers looked at a wide range of factors—age, muscle strength, muscle mass, hormone levels, medical conditions, and marital status—and their association with the metabolic syndrome. They found that muscle mass and strength were strong protective factors against the metabolic syndrome. Their research also suggested that a substantial proportion of metabolic syndrome cases could be prevented with a strength-training program.

A study from a Finnish researcher published in a 2011 issue of *Advances in Preventive Medicine* gets more specific about the benefits of strength training. It notes that resistance training has a favorable effect on metabolic syndrome because it decreases abdominal fat, enhances insulin sensitivity, improves glucose tolerance, and reduces blood pressure values. The researcher concludes, "Resistance training is probably the most effective measure to prevent and treat sarcopenia." Because the Quickie Rev Up incorporates a form of resistance training, it will help you develop the lean muscle that fights the Shrinking Muscle Syndrome and the conditions associated with it.

Unfortunate Dangers of Typical Diets…and the Overnight Diet Solution

	Early Death	Heart Disease	Type 2 Diabetes	Cancer	Kidney Problems	Moodiness / Depression	Malnutrition	Constipation	Bad Breath	"Diet Flu"
Typical	A 2010 study found that a low-carb diet rich in animal foods was associated with a 23 percent increase in mortality from all causes.	Some low-carb diets with high-fat content and a lack of dietary fiber contribute to cardiac risk factors, including high cholesterol.	The muscle loss that can occur with popular diets contributes to insulin resistance, which is a precursor to diabetes.	Low-fiber, high-fat, and low-carb diets may raise the risk of cancer.	Diets that tell you to eat only protein for any amount of time have been linked to kidney stones and other kidney problems.	Very low-calorie diets can make you feel light-headed, mentally foggy, and anxious. Low-carb diets can reduce serotonin levels, which can lead to blue moods.	Diets that encourage you to cut back on entire food groups or even limit variety can lead to deficiencies in vitamins, minerals, and other micronutrients.	Constipation is a common complaint among dieters following low-carb eating plans and can be directly attributed to a lack of fiber in the diet.	Low-carb diets and no-carb diets can cause embarrassing bad breath.	Severe carbohydrate restriction causes withdrawal symptoms that mimic the flu, including headache, nausea, fatigue, and an inability to concentrate.

The Overnight Diet Solution	Research shows that periodically enjoying a day like the 1-Day Power Up promotes a longer lifespan. Studies show that a high-protein diet rich in vegetables similar to the 6-Day Fuel Up is associated with a 20 percent reduced risk of death from all causes.	By focusing on lean carbs that are high in fiber, the Overnight Diet helps protect your heart. 2007 research shows that routinely following a day like the 1-Day Power Up accounted for a 40 percent reduced risk for heart disease.	The synergy created by the Overnight Diet is the ideal recipe for reducing your risk for developing type 2 diabetes, and it could be your ticket to reversing the disease.	This diet is overflowing with high-fiber, high-antioxidant, cancer-fighting foods. Research shows that high-fiber diets reduce the risk for colorectal cancer and that eating more fruits and vegetables reduces the risk for all types of cancer.	This diet is high in protein, but it is also high in fiber, which helps kidneys flush protein out of the body and maintain optimal function.	Abundant food on this diet prevents hunger, which cuts out the anxious feelings, light-headedness, and mental fog. Lean carbs encourage serotonin production, which is associated with more stable moods.	A wide variety of nutrient-dense foods from all food groups prevents any nutritional deficiencies.	High-fiber foods will keep your digestive tract moving smoothly.	Eating good-for-you lean carbs promotes weight loss and naturally fresh breath.	Whole grains and unlimited fruits and vegetables help make you feel great right from the start.

How to Use This Book

In the remainder of this book, you'll find everything you need to implement the Overnight Diet into your daily life. Part II lays out the basic guidelines of the program and shows you how to find your DPR, which is a critical component of this plan. In Part III, you'll find dozens of quick-fix recipes and a 28-day meal plan to help you get started. Part IV reveals the secrets to sticking to the diet wherever life takes you: on vacation, out with friends, or grabbing food on the go. And in the final chapter, you'll discover how to modify the diet after you've reached your goal weight, so you can maintain your weight loss for good.

PART II

THE OVERNIGHT DIET IN ACTION

CHAPTER 3

1-Day Power Up

On the 1-Day Power Up, you'll be enjoying a day of feasting on refreshing, invigorating, jumbo smoothies—Banana Latte, Piña Colada Island, or Enchanted Blueberry anyone? And you'll be doing this on a weekly basis until you reach your goal weight. There is one important caveat: As powerful and beneficial as the 1-Day Power Up is, don't do it more than once a week. Years of development and testing on thousands of patients have shown that once a week provides the optimal conditions to maximize its effectiveness.

The 1-Day Power Up was developed after patients at the Nutrition and Weight Management Center at Boston Medical Center kept complaining that they couldn't make it through those long, drawn-out initiation phases on other diets that required them to stick to short lists of approved foods for weeks or even months. "Isn't there a faster way to lose weight?" asked Amy, a twenty-seven-year-old freelance graphic designer who had just gotten divorced and wanted to lose 15 pounds before jumping back into the dating pool. Amy grumbled that she could never make it through those ultra-restrictive start-up periods and always ended up giving up too soon. Amy's story is common. Maybe you've caught yourself saying the same thing, too.

Decades of research show that taking a periodic break from solid food can safely produce the rapid weight loss Amy and other patients were looking for. This was the inspiration to enlist the help of lead nutritionist Diana Cullum-Dugan to create something so delicious

45

that people would actually look forward to it. The 1-Day Power Up isn't a day of deprivation, but rather a different kind of feast day. Twenty-five years of experience and knowledge about rapid weight loss, optimal nutrition, and muscle maintenance went into the development of a menu of rich, creamy smoothies packed with protein, fiber, and nutrients—not to mention lip-smacking ingredients like chocolate syrup, strawberries, and yogurt.

But would patients like Amy like them? Would they be able to get through the whole day without feeling hungry or giving up? The science showed that metabolically, when combined with the 6-Day Fuel Up, it could do exactly what my patients were asking for, but how would it work in real life? The 1-Day Power Up smoothies were put to the test, and what do you know? The patients couldn't stop raving about them. Amy told me she didn't feel hungry, and when she combined them with the 6-Day Fuel Up, she lost the 15 pounds fast enough to feel confident about dating again. She loved the smoothies. And you will, too.

At first, the idea of a smoothie feast day once a week may seem a bit drastic to you. That's understandable. After all, our society, the food industry, and many diet books force-feed us on the notion that we should be grazing constantly throughout the day. Rest assured that humans have been regularly taking breaks from solid food for thousands of years. Consider that even today, almost every major religion encourages this practice at certain times of the week, month, or year. Millions of people take a break from their usual fare for specific periods of time for religious or other reasons. Did you know that First Lady Michelle Obama routinely enjoys a modified two-day food break? That's right. The First Lady, who has made it her mission to fight obesity in America, told *Ladies' Home Journal* that she likes to take a periodic break from her regular meals to cleanse her palate and reduce cravings. And of course, remember Caveman Joe and Cavewoman Jane, who thrived even when they were looking for their next meal.

The human body is designed to work extremely efficiently during this period. It's when the body taps into its stores and burns them for fuel. Each and every one of us already engages in this practice on a daily basis—it's just that we typically do it at night while we're sleeping and in between meals.

Besides, with three jumbo smoothies that include *real foods*, this is not your typical "juice day." It's a veritable feast with a wide variety of rich, tasty drinks, including sweet smoothies such as Orange Zest, Mexican Chocolate Banana Swirl, and Tropical Medley; savory smoothies such as Kale Margarita; and veggie-packed "green" smoothies such as Green Machine. Some of them are so big, you probably won't be able to finish them in one sitting, which means you'll have enough left over for a tasty snack later in the day. And when you wake up the next morning and hop on that scale, you'll be amazed how easy weight loss can be.

Get Started Guidelines for Your 1-Day Power Up

Getting started with your 1-Day Power Up is such a breeze you'll be on the road to overnight weight loss in no time. Here's how you do it.

Important! If you have kidney disease or diabetes, check with your physician before starting the 1-Day Power Up.

Blender Basics

You'll be making three smoothies a day on a weekly basis, and since you may be using frozen fruit or ice in many of them, it's a good idea to choose a durable blender with a strong blade. The top blender on the market is the Vitamix, which offers professional strength, but is pricey at about $500. The Omni blender is another high-performance option that runs about $250. If you don't like a noisy blender, the Omni is a great option because it is quieter than most. If budget is important, Ninja offers several good models for less than $100. You can find all of these blenders and many more online.

If you're always on the run, look for single-serving blenders that allow you to "blend and go." With these space-saving devices, you can just pop off the top, which looks like a glass or sports bottle, and take it with you. Some blenders are so compact you can fit them into an overnight bag if you're going on vacation or out of town on business. Although convenient, these types of blenders may not have a very sturdy blade. This means you may have to introduce ice, frozen foods, and denser fruits and veggies little by little to avoid problems, such as the blender grinding to a halt or the blade breaking. With all blenders, you can ensure smoother blending by introducing fruits and veggies in order of density, going from the densest, such as carrots, to the lightest, such as spinach. If you're on the go and don't have access to a blender, don't worry. In Chapter 10, you'll find some tricks you can use to modify the recipes on the road.

Whichever blender you choose, be sure to retain the skin of the fruits (except for inedible skins such as banana peels) and veggies you use. A lot of the health-promoting, disease-fighting nutrients in produce are found in the skin. Plus, the skin and pulp contain all that good-for-you fiber, which is part of what helps keep you feeling full for hours, keeps your digestive system moving, and promotes good health.

Because it *is* so important that you get this fiber in your smoothies, it is recommended that you avoid using juicers for the 1-Day Power Up. Juicers have gained popularity as a weight-loss tool, but they squeeze out the juice from fruits and vegetables, eliminating the fiber.

Making the 1-Day Power Up Smoothies

If you're one of those people who like the ease of following goof-proof instructions, then by all means stick to using the smoothie recipes in Chapter 7. But if you prefer to get a little adventurous, you'll enjoy the option to create your own smoothies using the "Mix 'n' Match Smoothie Chart" (Appendix A, page 279). That's what Nathalie, a seventeen-year-old high school student, does. When

Nathalie started putting on a lot of weight following puberty, she tried dieting but would get bored with the lack of variety. When she learned that she could create her own smoothies for the 1-Day Power Up, she loved the idea and couldn't wait to start whipping up her own concoctions.

One day, she was trying out a new combo when a couple of her high school friends (who *weren't* dieting) stopped by to see her. She gave them a sample of her smoothie, and they absolutely loved it and asked for more. Now they come over each week on Nathalie's smoothie day as her official "taste testers." Together, they've come up with about thirty mixtures of their own. Nathalie, by the way, has lost 33 pounds and is now at a healthy weight, but still puts her smoothie day into practice.

If you want to create your own smoothies, just follow the easy steps here and use the "Mix 'n' Match Smoothie Chart" (Appendix A, page 279).

1. Choose 1 protein.
2. Choose 1 liquid.
3. Choose up to 2 fruits.
4. Choose up to 3 veggies.
5. Choose up to 2 add-ins (optional).
6. Choose 1 each of as many freebies as you would like (optional).
7. Throw them all into a blender and voilà!

If the thought of taking even a couple of minutes to whip up a delicious smoothie seems too time-consuming, or if you're on the road with no blender in sight, you have yet another option. You can grab my premixed blend that I developed for the Overnight Diet, called Physicians Protein Smoothies. It already includes everything you would throw in the blender, but in a convenient all-natural powder form that comes in a variety of flavors. Just add water, shake, and ta-da! You've got a flavored smoothie packed with 20 grams of a proprietary whey-casein protein blend that also includes 5 grams of dietary fiber, plus a host of other ingredients designed to increase satiety, facilitate weight loss, and taste great. You can find Physicians Protein Smoothies in stores that carry healthy foods and on the Overnight Diet website (OvernightDiet.org).

Whether you make your own blend, use the recipes provided, or grab a Physicians Protein Smoothie, these smoothies are delicious. Let's break down what these creative concoctions are made up of.

1-Day Power Up Smoothie Ingredients

Protein. Adding protein to your smoothies is essential for success on the Overnight Diet and packs a powerful punch—minimizing hunger throughout the day and fueling all-important lean muscle so you can boost metabolism, start burning fat faster, and avoid the Shrinking Muscle Syndrome. The protein in these smoothies comes from either protein powder or fat-free Greek yogurt.

The 411 on Protein Powders

Protein powders are a powerful way to pump up your protein intake on your smoothie feast day. These are derived from a number of sources and come in such a huge variety of flavors that you're sure to find one you'll love. But be aware that some powders contain gobs of sweeteners, so be sure to check the sugar content on the nutrition label and choose one with fewer than 2 grams of sugar per serving. With a dizzying array of products on the market, it can seem a bit confusing, but don't worry, the homework has already been done for you.

Through my scientific research and twenty-five years of practicing as a weight-loss doctor, I have discovered that the blending of whey protein isolate and casein protein powders provides the best protein option for fast, healthy, permanent weight loss. That is why I created the Physicians Protein Smoothies Base Mix. This specially formulated blend of whey and casein results in a short burst of proteins (from the whey) that makes you feel full as soon as you drink your smoothie. However, the effect of whey doesn't last long, so I added casein, which starts slowly but keeps you feeling full for longer, creating the most effective blend. You can also blend your own whey-casein protein powder at home! Simply purchase both a whey and a casein protein powder individually and create a 50:50 mix of each for use in your smoothies.

However, it is not necessary to use my Physicians Protein Smoothies Base Mix or mix your own whey-casein blend. There are many other good protein powders on the market. Just be sure to read the label carefully to ensure that your protein powder has approximately 20 grams of protein per serving. Be sure no more than 5 grams of sugar are added, and review all added ingredients.

Get the Skinny on the Science

Making the Case for Adding Omega-3 to Your Smoothies There is a growing body of evidence suggesting that increasing your intake of omega-3 fatty acids can reduce body weight and body fat if you're overweight or obese. Not only that, but omega-3 fatty acids can also reduce post-meal hunger, which means they can help keep your stomach from growling in between smoothies. Additional research points to a synergistic effect when you increase consumption of omega-3 fatty acids and engage in exercise—increasing the formation of lean muscle and bypassing the storage of excess calories in adipose tissue. That's all great, but who wants to put foul-tasting liquid omega-3 supplements into a smoothie? A better alternative is flaxseed, the richest source of the plant-based omega-3 fatty acid alpha-linolenic acid, which has a mild nutty flavor that tastes great in smoothies. That's why you'll find flaxseeds in several of the smoothie recipes, as well as in the Physicians Protein Smoothies and the Physicians Protein Smoothies Base Mix.

Vegan-Friendly Protein Powders

Soy protein powders are known for their antioxidant powers and are as digestible as other sources of protein. Soy protein is considered a complete protein as it provides all the amino acids necessary for nutrition. If you are vegan, soy protein is an affordable and popular vegetable-source protein powder. However, if you suffer from multiple food allergies or a thyroid problem, please be aware that soy is a common allergen.

If you are looking for another vegetable-source protein powder, you can try rice protein powder. However, rice protein lacks two essential amino acids (lycine and threonine) and is, therefore, nutritionally incomplete. This makes rice protein an unsafe sole source of protein, as your body requires all the essential amino acids for optimal system function. To create a complete protein, combine with pea protein in a 50:50 blend.

Pea protein powder is a low-calorie, nutrient-dense protein powder option. Silky smooth and easily blended, this protein powder is a great choice for those who suffer from lactose intolerance. However, be aware that, as with rice protein, it is nutritionally incomplete and lacking essential amino acids. For my vegan friends, you can blend pea protein powder with brown rice protein powder to achieve a nutritionally complete, plant-based protein powder that will contain all the essential amino acids.

Hempseed protein powder contains both essential and nonessential amino acids, as well as iron, calcium, and omega-3 fatty acids. However, hempseed may be digested and absorbed to varying degrees. Make sure to look for unhulled hempseed, which has a higher digestibility rate (66 percent) than other hempseed proteins.

While there are many fabulous vegetable-source protein powders on the market, animal-source protein powders are nutritionally superior.

Dairy-Based Protein Powders

Whey protein is fast digesting, which means it is emptied from the stomach quickly, providing a superior effect on muscle protein balance. This is an advantage after a workout or in the morning but a disadvantage for keeping you feeling full until your next meal. It is a complete food and provides both essential and nonessential amino acids. However, whey protein does contain lactose, which is an important consideration for those who cannot tolerate it. An alternative to using whey protein is to choose whey protein isolate, which has minimal amounts of lactose.

Casein, the most abundant protein in milk, has a slower rate of digestion, and results in a slow but steady release of amino acids into circulation. However, like whey, it contains lactose and can cause bloating in those who may be allergic. It sometimes has a high sodium content, so check the label before purchasing.

Goat whey protein powder is another option. Unlike whey protein powder from cow's milk, this type of whey is 15 to 20 percent protein, with the rest being carbs. Therefore, it's not the greatest protein supplement to use for gaining muscle. However, goat whey protein powder is very high in minerals, and easy to digest.

Egg white protein powder contains all the essential amino acids your body needs and remains low in fat and calories. However, it contains cholesterol and may cause gas and bloating in some individuals. It tends to be a bit pricier than other protein powders and should be avoided if you have allergy concerns.

If you decide to forgo protein powder entirely, you have the option of getting that essential protein by adding in one cup of nonfat, plain Greek yogurt to your smoothies. Something to keep in mind is that Greek yogurt contains lower levels of calcium than other kinds of yogurt, a drawback of the straining process. Depending on your preference, the taste of Greek yogurt can be an advantage or a disadvantage.

If your taste buds absolutely refuse to go Greek, go ahead and find a yogurt you like. Just make sure to choose a fat-free or 1% low-fat variety that is low in sugar (12 grams or less per 6-ounce serving), which means skipping the kind that has the fruit at the bottom. And remember that you may also need to toss in some protein powder to make up for the lower amount of protein in other yogurts.

Look for Yogurt with Live Cultures

If you want to maintain a healthy digestive system, opt for yogurt that contains live cultures. These products will have the words "Live and Active Cultures" on the package. This means the yogurt is a great source of "good" bacteria, known as probiotics, which help balance the natural bacteria in your intestines. The most common probiotic found in yogurt is Lactobacillus acidophilus. Probiotics may help reduce gas, diarrhea, cramping, and the symptoms of irritable bowel syndrome. There is also some evidence that they may prevent or minimize vaginal yeast infections as well as cold and flu symptoms.

Liquid. In making your smoothies, you can use fat-free milk, your favorite fat-free or low-fat dairy-free alternative, tasty juice, or just water, as well as ice—it's up to you. If you opt for juice, use less than if you were using the other liquids. Juice packs more calories and sugar without any protein or any of the heart-healthy fiber you get when eating the whole fruit.

Dairy-Free Options

If you have problems digesting milk or you would just like to try an alternative to milk, there are a lot of great options, including:

Soy milk. Many people are drinking soy milk for its health benefits. Derived from soybeans, it is high in protein and contains more fiber than regular milk. It also contains soy isoflavones, which have been linked to reducing the risk for heart disease, cancer, and osteoporosis. It has also been found to reduce menopause symptoms in some women. Cholesterol-free and low in saturated fat, soy milk also provides vitamin D and calcium.

Almond milk. Almond milk is becoming more and more popular, and there are more brands and more varieties—including vanilla and chocolate!—on grocery store shelves. The fact that it is low in calories, low in cholesterol, low in sodium, and low in sugar explains part of its appeal. Add in healthy doses of calcium, vitamin D, vitamin E, and vitamin A, and it's easy to see why people are giving almond milk a try. When choosing almond milk, opt for an unsweetened variety.

Coconut milk. Coconuts and coconut milk were once considered diet disasters because they contain natural saturated fats. But emerging research has found that the type of saturated fat in coconuts is rapidly used as energy rather than being stored as fat. Even so, choose light coconut milk rather than the full-fat version. It contains vitamins and minerals that support the immune system. Note that coconut milk and coconut water are *not* one and the same. Coconut milk is derived from squeezing the flesh of the coconut. The clear liquid that drains from the fruit is coconut water. If you want to use coconut water, look for brands that are unsweetened.

Get the Skinny on the Science

Why the Fat in Coconut Milk Won't Make You Fat Not all saturated fat is created equal. Coconuts and coconut milk are rich in medium-chain fatty acids (MCFAs), a type of saturated fat that is quickly metabolized by the liver. This means the body rapidly burns it as fuel rather than sending it to your fat cells for storage. Compare that to long-chain fatty acids (LCFAs), which are the saturated fats typically found in meats and dairy products. Research on animals has shown that LCFAs are more likely to wind up as fat on the body. In a few small human studies, people eating a diet rich in MCFAs had higher metabolism than those consuming LCFAs.

Fruit. You can use fresh fruits, canned fruits, or frozen fruits (unsweetened). If you use canned fruits, make sure the fruit is canned in its own juice rather than in syrup and always drain the juice first. Filled with disease-fighting antioxidants, fruits are also a good source of fiber, which helps you feel full longer so you don't get the munchies 20 minutes after you finish your smoothie. On the Overnight Diet, *all* fruits are acceptable.

Nonstarchy veggies. Use fresh veggies whenever possible, but you can also use frozen or canned veggies in a pinch. Want to know one of the coolest things about sneaking veggies into smoothies? Sure, they pack a powerful nutrition punch while adding healthy fiber—but the best thing is you can't even taste them! Even if you've never been a big fan of spinach or kale, you don't have to worry— they won't ruin the flavor for you!

They didn't bother Emily, a college student who at twenty-three years of age had already successfully lost 18 pounds, but she had hit a plateau and just couldn't get rid of those last 10 pounds. When she heard about the 1-Day Power Up and how it helps break through plateaus, she was eager to try it. Fortunately, she showed up at the Nutrition and Weight Management Center at Boston Medical Center on a day when several smoothies were being subjected to a taste test. Emily was told she could pick one to try. "I love chocolate," she said, and zeroed in on the Spa Crazy Chocolate Smoothie (page 146). After a few sips, Emily gave it a big thumbs-up. "What's in it?" When she saw the list of ingredients, which included spinach, Emily just about fell out of her chair. "You're kidding me! There's no way this can have spinach in it. I *hate* spinach," she said.

As you'll discover, adding veggies is a sneaky way to get more fiber without significantly altering the taste of the smoothie. As for Emily, she now throws in handfuls of spinach knowing she'll get lots of great nutrients without having to taste it. And she adds, "I wish my mom would have been smart enough to give me my veggies this way."

Add-Ins (optional). The same way those frozen yogurt shops let you perfect your own creation with a wide array of toppings, here's where you can really have some fun with your smoothies. Think chocolate syrup, peanut butter, blackstrap molasses, and more! Some of the Add-Ins may seem a little out of the ordinary to you, but they are delicious and all of them boast health benefits. But just as toppings are optional at those frozen yogurt shops, so are Add-Ins; it's completely up to you whether to include them or not.

Freebies (optional). This is where you will find flavorings, spices, sugar substitutes, and other goodies that can really make your smoothie your own. Love cinnamon or nutmeg for a holiday-themed smoothie? Sprinkle away! Want to blend vanilla extract with an orange to create a smoothie that reminds you of a Creamsicle? Go right ahead. Love iced coffee drinks? Try adding brewed coffee to create a mocha latte smoothie. It's up to you.

Spice Up Your Smoothies with a Little (or a Lot) of Flavor

Turning your smoothies into fun, fanciful creations is easy. Flavorings and extracts as well as spices from your kitchen cupboards can transform an ordinary smoothie into something extraordinary. With all of these, a little goes a long way; you only need to use a small amount to get a big taste—¼ to ½ teaspoon of spices and ¼ to 1 teaspoon of flavorings and extracts. The latter may contain calories and sweeteners, but because you'll be using such small doses, the amounts are negligible. In terms of flavorings and extracts, you can use traditional ones such as vanilla, chocolate, orange, lemon, or lime. But if you really want to get creative, there are many unique tasty flavors you can find. The same goes for spices. Check the "Smoothie Flavorings and Extracts" list (Appendix A, page 281) and the "Smoothie Spices" list (Appendix A, page 281) for ideas. If you can't find the ones you want in your local grocery store, you can find a wide selection online.

Sweet Success

Two no-calorie sweeteners that are recommended on the Overnight Diet are Truvia, which is made with stevia, and Splenda, which is also known as sucralose. You can find Truvia and Splenda in just about any grocery store or market. Stevia is just catching on as a sugar substitute. If you can't find it in your local market, you can order it online. It comes in both a powder form and in a variety of guilt-free liquid flavors, including chocolate, cinnamon, English toffee, grape, hazelnut, lemon, peppermint, root beer, and vanilla.

Revel in an R&R Day

When you get started on the Overnight Diet, you'll first choose one day of the week to be your weekly 1-Day Power Up day. Many people choose Sunday because they don't have to work and are at home, where they have all their smoothie ingredients at hand and can just focus on relaxing (you'll find more information about the "rest and relaxation" part of this day later in this chapter). Pick the day that will work best for you consistently—it doesn't matter which day that is.

Another reason people love the 1-Day Power Up so much is because in addition to jump-starting the metabolic processes that induce overnight weight loss, it also acts as a wind-down "R&R day." That's right, you have permission to take a break from physical activity—if you want to—and luxuriate in a day of rest and relaxation. Think of how a plug-in hybrid electric car is charged while in the "off" mode, restoring the energy it spent on its last trip and juicing up for its next outing. That's what this transitional and transformational day can do for you: rejuvenate and recharge.

On the very first day you start the Overnight Diet, the 1-Day Power Up will be doing just that—powering up your body for the coming week. On subsequent 1-Day Power Up days, you will not only be charging up for the coming week, but also taking a breather from the previous week's 6-Day Fuel Up. Think of the R&R aspect of this day like a spa day when you get to pamper yourself and enjoy some well-deserved "me time." Do your best to take it easy. Here are some of the ways my weight-loss patients choose to unwind:

"My husband gives me a nice neck-and-shoulder massage in the evening. It's so relaxing."

"I turn on some calming music while I'm going about my day."

"I sit on the couch and watch football."

"I cozy up in my favorite chair and read a book."

"I like to do some gentle stretching."

"I take a nap in the afternoon. What a luxury!"

"I write in my journal."

"I spend time with friends."

Taking a respite from your hectic life can do wonders for your moods and help you de-stress, which is yet another way the 1-Day Power Up works to encourage weight loss. Mountains of scientific evidence have identified a strong link between stress and weight gain, and in particular with an increase in belly fat. In fact, women who have slender arms, legs, and hips but fat around the abdomen have been found to have high levels of the stress hormone cortisol. Feeling frazzled day in and day out raises levels of cortisol, which wreaks havoc on your weight. It can slow your metabolism, cause your body to store fat around the abdominal organs, affect your blood sugar levels, reduce levels of the body's muscle-building hormones, and increase cravings. To put it simply, stress leads to weight gain, emotional eating, and the Shrinking Muscle Syndrome. Taking advantage of the weekly 1-Day Power Up to relax and rejuvenate can help reverse this process.

Just ask Karen, a forty-year-old working mother of three, who had about 30 pounds to lose. Karen was so busy with her job, housework, and shuttling her kids to and from school and activities that she felt stressed all the time. She wanted to lose weight but she didn't have a lot of time to devote to a diet with a bunch of complicated recipes or a lengthy initiation phase. She wanted a quick and easy method to lose weight, and she wanted fast results…like tomorrow! She loved the idea of overnight weight loss that lasts, and was eager to get started.

Fast-forward to one of her follow-up appointments, and Karen was thrilled that she was quickly zeroing in on her goal. That's not unusual on this diet, but then Karen explained how the 1-Day Power Up had literally changed her life.

Get the Skinny on the Science

De-stress to Weigh Less Reducing stress is one of the key ingredients for weight loss, according to a study appearing in a 2011 issue of the *International Journal of Obesity*. A team of scientists from Kaiser Permanente Center for Health Research enlisted almost 500 participants and asked them to lose at least 10 pounds in 6 months. The volunteers were also asked to report on their stress levels, in addition to their sleep habits, moods, and more. The results showed that participants with the lowest stress levels who got at least 6 but not more than 8 hours of sleep were the most likely to lose at least 10 pounds. In fact, they were twice as likely to have lost 10 or more pounds than the people who reported the highest stress levels and got less than 6 hours of shut-eye on a regular basis.

Karen said that the weekly R&R day had helped her learn how to relax and de-stress. Just taking some time out for herself on that one day per week allowed her to recharge her batteries so she didn't feel so run-down and crazed all the time. "I think I had forgotten how to relax and pamper myself," she said. "And I really needed to rediscover that."

But that's not all. The 1-Day Power Up also made her completely reevaluate her relationship with food. She quickly realized that she had been using food as a way to self-soothe—to calm her when she felt stressed; to boost her mood when she felt sad, mad, or anxious; and to give her something to do when she was bored. It was also a form of entertainment for her. Every family outing revolved around food—going out to dinner, stopping for a celebratory dessert after one of the kid's soccer matches, filling up on popcorn and soda at the movies. Every get-together with her girlfriends, such as her monthly book group meeting, involved lots of fattening foods or cocktails, and sometimes both. Every work event she attended turned into a food foray, too.

"It was like I couldn't survive more than an hour without eating something," Karen said. "I was convinced that I was going to be starving on the 1-Day Power Up. But when I actually tried it, I wasn't hungry at all in between my smoothies. I couldn't believe it. Throughout the rest of the week, I started paying attention to the times when I would feel hungry, and it finally dawned on me that most of the time when I would eat, it rarely had anything to do with actually being hungry. That was an eye-opener for me."

Tales of the Measuring Tape

"I don't cook so I love the smoothie day. It's so easy, even I can do it."
—Joseph, 56, lost 47 pounds

A lot of people experience this kind of breakthrough just by practicing the 1-Day Power Up. Don't worry, though. With this diet, you don't have to do any deep soul-searching about the emotional reasons *why* you overeat; you don't have to keep a food diary; and you don't have to start journaling your every thought and emotion. However, gaining an awareness of your appetite can help you get in tune with your body's hunger and satiety signals. Engaging in some simple mindful eating habits is one way to do so. Here are a few tips:

- Before you eat, ask yourself, "Am I really hungry?"
- Sit down to eat your meals or drink your smoothies as opposed to standing.
- Don't watch TV, read the newspaper, or check your e-mail while eating.
- Savor your food—or your smoothie—rather than wolfing it down.
- Eat as if others were watching you. In public, you probably wouldn't stuff your face.
- Eat—or drink—until you are satisfied. On a scale of 1 to 10, 1 being ravenous and 10 being post–Thanksgiving dinner full, aim for a 7 (not still hungry, but not stuffed either).

The 1-Day Power Up can go a long way toward changing the way you eat—for the better! It helped Karen change some of the food habits that were contributing to those 30 extra pounds she had been carrying around. "At first, I thought I couldn't go to my book group meeting because it was my smoothie day. That if I wasn't going to partake in the big plate of cookies we always ate, I somehow wasn't participating in the group. But then I realized how stupid that thought was. Why couldn't I just take my smoothie with me to the book group?"

So Karen showed up one night to her book group with one of her own smoothie creations—a tropical concoction with a banana-flavored protein powder, light coconut milk, and mango. Her friends were so impressed with her new slimmed-down appearance that they wanted to know what she was drinking and asked for the recipe. So the next time she hosted the book group, Karen decided to make smoothies instead of putting out the usual spread of cookies. Her friends loved it! Now their book group night has become a smoothie night. And some of the other women in the group have started following the Overnight Diet and losing weight with Karen.

The simple yet powerful realization that she didn't have to be a slave to her old eating habits at the book group led to other lifestyle changes for Karen, which, when combined with her 1-Day Power Up and 6-Day Fuel Up, sparked even speedier weight loss. And it has helped her keep that weight off. Karen reached her goal weight three years ago, and hasn't gained a pound since.

Tales of the Measuring Tape

"Having an R&R day is the best. Carving out a day of 'me' time each Sunday allows my body, and my mind, to get the rest it needs. Then when Monday comes along, I feel energized and ready to go for the week."

—Nina, age 31, lost 21 pounds and has kept it off for 19 months

---

Power Up and Prep

The 1-Day Power Up also serves as an ideal prep day to get ready for the upcoming 6-Day Fuel Up. It's a great time to review the meal plan for the coming week, to ensure that your fridge is stocked with the good-for-you foods you will be eating on the 6-Day Fuel Up, to prep snacks so you can just grab and go, and to prepare any recipes that might taste better if made a day or two before consuming them. That way, when you come home from work in the evenings—voilà!—everything's all ready to go. You don't have to worry about what you're going to make, and you don't have to run to the store for ingredients you don't have.

CHAPTER 4

6-Day Fuel Up

If you have already completed your 1-Day Power Up, congratulations! You are up to 2 pounds lighter, and you have revved up your body's fat-burning process. The next six days are the key to keeping up the momentum so you can continue to burn fat and lose up to 9 pounds in the first week.

As we have discussed, the foundation of the 6-Day Fuel Up lies in a diet plan first used in a medical setting. But for a diet to be effective long-term, it can't just produce results in the lab or in a medically supervised setting. It has to work in the crazy reality we call life, where on some days you have mere minutes to get the entire family fed and out the door in the morning and then you have just 15 minutes to whip up dinner in the evening. Rest assured, the 6-Day Fuel Up has been developed with real people in mind and has been engineered to produce maximum results safely *and* be easy enough to follow that it works in the real world, without any necessary doctor supervision.

You've already learned how it works together with the 1-Day Power Up to maintain fat burning at a high level, how it contributes to the production of lean muscle, and how it promotes optimal health. But now you're about to discover why it will be a breeze for you to follow:

You won't go hungry. The foods you will be eating during these six days have been shown to provide the greatest levels of satiety. This means they will keep you feeling full the longest. Plus, if you do get the munchies, you can choose from lots of grab-and-go snacks...guilt free!

You won't feel deprived. Many diets bombard you with endless lists of foods to avoid, leaving you with extremely limited choices. When there's next to nothing that you are allowed to eat, it increases the likelihood that you will give up long before you get the results you want. On the Overnight Diet, you won't have that problem. The focus of the 6-Day Fuel Up is on feeding the muscles with adequate protein and fueling the body with great-tasting, good-for-you foods that will result in rapid fat loss, *not* deprivation. There is an abundance of delicious foods, and no food group is off limits; you won't even feel like you're dieting. Instead of telling you what to take away, the Overnight Diet lets you add to your plate with unlimited veggies and fruits—a veritable bottomless buffet.

Let's meet Ed here. At fifty-one, Ed loved Mexican food, spicy chili, and double-decker burgers, all of which contributed to the extra 30 pounds of fat he had been carrying around for about twenty years. To trim down, Ed would periodically try some sort of crash diet. He would typically lose about 10 pounds pretty quickly, but he always felt as if he was starving to death, and he was so deprived of all the foods he loved that he could never stick with these drastic plans. After a couple of weeks, he would usually chuck the whole plan out the window and go on a week-long binge, gaining back all 10 pounds...and a couple more.

When he tried the Overnight Diet, he was amazed that he could eat so much food and so many of the foods he loved—with a healthy twist—and still lose weight. He didn't feel deprived so he found it easy to stay on the plan. He eventually lost those 30 pounds and has kept them off for more than two years. Check out the box below to see what Ed would eat on a typical day on the 6-Day Fuel Up.

Ed's 6-Day Fuel Up Meals

Breakfast: Breakfast Tacos (with eggs, Cheddar cheese, spinach, and salsa on corn tortillas), an orange, and coffee

Snack: Baked Cinnamon Apple

Lunch: Beefy Mushroom Burger and an apple

Snack: Veggies with Avocado Corn Salsa
Dinner: Spicy Chicken and White Bean Chili, Baked Parmesan
  Tomatoes, and a glass of Pinot Noir
Dessert: Grandma's Low-Fat Chocolate Pudding
Snack: Blueberries

You won't get bored. With more than 100 lip-smacking foods you can eat right from the start, you won't be forced to eat the same ho-hum fare day in and day out. Variety will keep you engaged and excited while you slim down.

Get the Skinny on the Science

Variety Is the Spice of a Healthy Life Diets that severely restrict the types of foods you can eat or that eliminate entire categories of food may be sabotaging your health, according to University of Arkansas researcher Peter Ungar, author of *Human Diet: Its Origin and Evolution.* Ungar points to evidence suggesting that humans evolved to consume a wider array of foods than any other species. And when it comes to our health, the wider, the better. So instead of narrowing your choices to a few select approved foods, it is better for your health to enjoy a wide variety of foods like you will on the Overnight Diet. It's guaranteed you'll like it better, too.

You'll love the flexibility. If you're running late, you will find foods and meals that you can simply grab on your way out the door. Or if you enjoy getting creative in the kitchen, you can experiment to your heart's content. You also don't have to worry about fitting meals into a rigid schedule. You don't have to eat breakfast at 7:38 a.m., a snack exactly two hours and twelve minutes later, lunch at 12:17 p.m., another snack exactly three hours and seven minutes later, and then dinner at 6:06 p.m. Life can get crazy, and a diet has to fit into your schedule in order for it to work long-term, so there is flexibility built into this plan.

You don't have to be an algebra whiz. Phew! You can forget about counting calories, adding up points, weighing every serving of food, calculating ratios of macronutrients to put on your plate, or figuring out percentages of your daily intake. There is only one number you need to know: your DPR, and the charts on pages 68–69 will do the calculating for you.

Get the Skinny on the Science

Easy Does It, Complicated Doesn't It may seem obvious, but diets that are more complicated, that involve a lot of rules and requirements, and that take up a lot of time are harder to stick with. That means that the more complicated a diet is, the more likely you are to give up on it without getting the weight-loss benefits you want. This insight comes from a 2010 study in *Appetite*, in which cognitive scientists from Indiana University and the Max Planck Institute for Human Development in Berlin compared how women fared on two very different diet plans. One diet involved very simple meal plans while the other required dieters to calculate every morsel of food they ate. The scientists found that the more complicated people thought their diet plan was, the faster they gave up on it.

There's no guesswork. At the Nutrition and Weight Management Center at Boston Medical Center, there is a food pantry stocked with fresh fruits and vegetables in addition to canned foods so patients can see firsthand what a healthy pantry looks like. On page 283, you'll find the Overnight Diet Shopping List to help you create your own Overnight Diet pantry. It's easier than you think.

Tales of the Measuring Tape

"I can't tell you how happy I am that I don't have to count calories!"
—Lynette, 31, lost 19 pounds

You'll love the simplicity. On the 6-Day Fuel Up, there are only four simple prescriptions to follow. They aren't time-consuming, they don't require any expensive equipment, and they don't involve complicated food combining. Just four clear, easy-to-follow, fat-blasting, weight-busting prescriptions. And if you follow these, you will see results…fast. Let's look more closely at each of them.

The R$_x$ for Faster Fat Loss

All you have to do is adhere to the following four simple prescriptions and you will be on your way to a whole new you, including a slimmer, trimmer, and stronger body.

Prescription 1: Meet your DPR every day.

Meeting your daily DPR is an indispensable component of the 6-Day Fuel Up. Getting adequate protein each day not only preserves lean muscle to boost metabolism and prevent the Shrinking Muscle Syndrome, but also prevents hunger pangs. As you have seen, protein rates high in terms of satiety, meaning it keeps you feeling full for hours. When you are eating the proper amount of protein, your stomach won't be grumbling. Here's how to find your DPR:

Daily Protein Requirement (DPR):
Ideal Weight (in kilograms) × 1.5 grams = DPR (in grams)

The first step is to convert your ideal weight from pounds to kilograms. But don't worry, the conversion and the math have already been calculated for you. Just find your ideal weight in pounds in the charts on pages 68 and 69. At the Nutrition and Weight Management Center at Boston Medical Center, a complex formula is used to determine each individual's ideal weight, but this has been simplified for you here. For women, ideal weight is 100 pounds for the first 5 feet in height and an additional 5 pounds for every inch over 5 feet; for men, it is 106 pounds for the first 5 feet in height and an additional 6 pounds for every inch over 5 feet. If you want to find your weight in kilograms, you can use the formula below. After you find your ideal weight on the chart, simply read across to find your DPR in grams.

Converting Pounds to Kilograms:
Ideal Weight (in pounds) ÷ 2.2 = Ideal Weight (in kilograms)

Keep reading across to find your DPR in ounces. Converting from grams to ounces is easy. There are about 7 grams of protein in every ounce of meat, poultry, or fish, so just take your DPR in grams and divide that number by 7 to get your DPR in ounces. That's already been done for you, too.

DPR in Ounces:
DPR (in grams) ÷ 7 = DPR (in ounces)

Remember, your DPR is the *minimum* amount of protein you need to consume *each day* on the Overnight Diet. Commit your

FIND YOUR DPR (FOR WOMEN)

Find your height on the left then read across to find your ideal weight and DPR in grams and ounces.

Height	Ideal Weight	DPR in Grams	DPR in Ounces
up to 5'4"	up to 120	82	12
5'5"	125	85	12
5'6"	130	89	13
5'7"	135	92	13
5'8"	140	95	14
5'9"	145	99	14
5'10"	150	102	15
5'11"	155	105	15
6'0"	160	109	16
6'1"	165	112	16
6'2"	170	116	17

FIND YOUR DPR (FOR MEN)

Find your height on the left then read across to find your ideal weight and DPR in grams and ounces.

Height	Ideal Weight	DPR in Grams	DPR in Ounces
up to 5′6″	up to 142	97	14
5′7″	148	101	14
5′8″	154	105	15
5′9″	160	109	16
5′10″	166	113	16
5′11″	172	117	17
6′0″	178	121	17
6′1″	184	125	18
6′2″	190	129	18
6′3″	196	133	19
6′4″	202	137	20
6′5″	208	141	20

DPR in grams and ounces to memory, or write the numbers down. There is one caveat, however: Even if your ideal weight is below 120 pounds, your minimum DPR will still be 82 grams, or 12 ounces if you're a woman; 97 grams or 14 ounces if you're a man. Eating less protein than that can be dangerous no matter how petite you are.

Here's an example of how this equation works. Let's say you are a 5-foot-9 male. According to the chart above, your ideal weight is 160 pounds. Just look across the chart to find your DPR in grams (109 grams) and your DPR in ounces (16 ounces). This means you would need to eat a *minimum* of 109 grams, or 16 ounces, of protein

Tales of the Measuring Tape

"I thought I was eating enough protein, but I guess I wasn't. Since I upped my protein intake, I've definitely noticed a difference in my body composition—less fat and more toned. I love it!"

—Leslie, lost 12 pounds and 2.5 inches off her waist

per day. Remember, this is just an example. You must determine your individual DPR to make the Overnight Diet work for you.

Getting adequate protein for your individual needs is a cornerstone of this program. It's what fuels your muscles and boosts metabolism. Getting the right type of protein is also important. In general, when it comes to protein, the leaner the better. On the 6-Day Fuel Up, you must meet your minimum DPR with the following lean protein sources: lean beef, lean pork, poultry, and fish; eggs and egg substitutes; soy products and meat alternatives; and protein powder.

Other protein sources do not count toward your DPR. This means that even though this eating plan recommends 2 servings daily of fat-free or low-fat (1%) dairy and up to 1 serving daily of legumes and pulses such as lentils, chickpeas, and black-eyed peas, the protein in these foods does not count toward your DPR. Why not? In addition to containing protein, these foods contain carbohydrates and natural sugars, which react differently in the body and do not provide the same level of muscle-preserving, fat-burning benefits compared to the more pure protein sources listed below. This is why these foods are limited to the number of servings indicated. Below is a list of lean protein options that are recommended for the 6-Day Fuel Up.

Protein Sources That Count Toward Your DPR for the 6-Day Fuel Up

Lean meats	beef, lamb, pork, veal
Lean game meats	bison, rabbit, venison
Fish	tuna, halibut, salmon, cod, canned fish in water, shellfish
Poultry	light meat chicken, turkey, pheasant, quail
Eggs	hard-boiled, soft-cooked, poached, pan-fried with nonstick cooking spray, egg whites, egg substitutes
Soy products and meat alternatives	tofu, tempeh, seitan, textured vegetable protein (TVP)
Protein powder	whey, soy, whey-casein blend, Physicians Protein Smoothies Base

Figuring out how much protein to eat to meet your DPR is easy if you're choosing beef, pork, fish, or poultry—1 ounce of these protein sources equals 1 ounce of protein toward your DPR. But what about eggs, tofu, and other sources? Use the following chart as a reference tool.

How Much Protein Equals 1 Ounce of Protein Toward Your DPR?

Protein Source	Protein Toward DPR
1 ounce lean beef	1 ounce
1 ounce lean pork	1 ounce
1 ounce fish	1 ounce
1 ounce poultry	1 ounce
1 large egg	1 ounce
2 large egg whites	1 ounce
¼ cup egg substitute	1 ounce
3 ounces tofu	1 ounce
1.5 ounces tempeh	1 ounce
1 ounce seitan	1 ounce
⅛ cup TVP	1 ounce
⅓ serving protein powder	Approximately 1 ounce (check label)

Just Say No: Higher-Fat Protein Sources
You should avoid higher-fat protein sources because dietary fats can be a contributing factor in insulin resistance and inflammation, both of which promote weight gain and obesity.

- **Higher-fat meats:** regular ground beef, prime grade or heavily marbled meats, spare ribs, goose, duck, wild game, organ meats
- **Processed meats:** bacon, sausage, corned beef, kielbasa, hot dogs, luncheon meats and cold cuts with more than 3 grams fat per ounce
- **Dairy:** whole milk, full-fat yogurt, full-fat cheeses, cream, whipped cream

Can I Do the Overnight Diet If I'm a Vegetarian?
Yes! It is easier than you might think to meet your DPR with soy products, meat alternatives, and eggs or egg substitutes. If you're a vegetarian or a vegan, you can replace poultry, pork, or beef in any meal in the meal plan or in the recipes with tofu, seitan, or tempeh. Another meat substitute is textured vegetable protein (TVP), which is made from dried soy protein. All you have to do is place equal parts TVP and boiling water into a measuring cup, wait 5 minutes, and it's ready to go. For meals that call for bacon or sausage, you can use veggie versions of these products, such as Morningstar Farms, which can be found in most supermarkets. In recipes that call for chicken or beef broth or stock, feel free to use vegetable broth or stock instead.

Prescription 2: Stick to lean carbs. You can enjoy a bottomless buffet of all-you-can-eat fruits and nonstarchy vegetables, up to 1 cup of starchy veggies, and 2–3 servings of whole grains absolutely guilt-free.

You should enjoy an abundant variety of lean carbs—high-fiber, heart-healthy, disease-fighting foods. Lean carbs are the good-for-you carbs that will *help* you lose the muffin top or love handles and keep them off. Remember, research shows that people who eat the most lean carbs are the least likely to be overweight or obese—but they must be the *right* carbs. It's time to stop feeling guilty for eating fruit or having a slice of whole-grain bread and start enjoying them again. Your body will thank you for it.

Savor all the fruits and nonstarchy vegetables you want from your bottomless buffet. When was the last time you got the green light to enjoy "all you can eat" of anything? Avoiding hunger pangs is essential when trying to lose weight; endless produce ensures that you will never go hungry. Think fruits and veggies are boring? "Spice Up Your Veggies" (Appendix B, page 288) and "Spice Up Your Fruit" (Appendix B, page 289) offer tips on how to turn ordinary produce into something extraordinary.

Does this mean you can't have *any* starchy veggies on the 6-Day

Fuel Up? No, it doesn't. Although your three snacks a day will be made up solely of fruits and nonstarchy veggies, your meals can include these as well as up to 1 cup of starchy veggies a day, including corn, potatoes, sweet potatoes, winter squash, yams, and yucca.

Did you know...

The new-look MyPlate, which replaced the old Food Pyramid, also places a major emphasis on fruits and vegetables. Amid the media storm surrounding the unveiling of the new food icon in 2011, First Lady Michelle Obama proclaimed that in the crusade against obesity, "As long as [plates are] half full of fruits and vegetables, and paired with lean proteins, whole grains, and low-fat dairy, we're golden." Sounds like she could have been talking about the 6-Day Fuel Up!

The fiber factor. Staving off hunger is only one of the reasons why this diet places such a strong emphasis on lean carbs, fruits, and vegetables. That high satiety factor is achieved in large part thanks to all the healthy fiber they contain. And fiber contributes to better health in a number of ways, which include:

- Reducing hunger
- Reducing cholesterol
- Reducing the risk for heart disease and stroke
- Reducing the risk for cancer
- Reducing the risk for type 2 diabetes
- Helping maintain optimal kidney function
- Improving bowel function

But remember, much of the fiber—as well as the vitamins and minerals—is found in the skin of the fruits and vegetables so eat them without peeling when possible. Of course, you have to peel bananas and oranges, but it's best to eat apples, pears, cucumbers, zucchini, and others with the skin on for a quick fiber boost.

Quick shopping tip for fruits and vegetables. Fresh produce makes great go-to snacks, but it can spoil if you don't eat it soon

enough. It's a good idea to keep canned and frozen fruits and vegetables in your pantry so you will always have them on hand. When
buying canned, choose fruits in water or in their own juices rather
than in syrup, and look for canned vegetables that aren't loaded with
sodium. With frozen foods, opt for fruits without added sugar and
vegetables without butter or cream sauces.

This plan is formulated to help you lose weight in a way that promotes good health rather than endangering it. There is a veritable
bounty of health benefits that come from eating fruits and vegetables.
Why are these foods such powerful disease fighters? Think of your
body for a moment like a big factory. Inside your factory, your cells—
which are like the employees on your production line—are hard at
work every moment of every day converting oxygen to energy. But
each time they do so, they create a by-product—molecules called free
radicals. Think of free radicals as Ninja assassins that race through your
body's factory damaging and destroying the equipment—proteins,
tissues, and genes. The work of these Ninja assassins is associated with
many diseases, including cancer and heart disease. To counterattack
the Ninja assassins, your body relies on an army of soldiers called antioxidants. Like superheroes, antioxidants neutralize the Ninjas so your
body's equipment can keep operating at full steam.

Where does your body get antioxidants? Fruits and vegetables!
Unfortunately, Americans eat only 59 percent of the daily recommended amount of vegetables and 42 percent of fruits. The Overnight
Diet aims to counteract this problem by encouraging you to eat abundant amounts of them, which help fight disease and keep your body in
peak condition. Plus, with dozens of fruits and vegetables from which
to choose, you will never get bored. The name of the game on this diet
is variety, not deprivation. Check out "The Overnight Diet Shopping
List" (Appendix B, page 283) to see the many fruits and vegetables
you can enjoy while burning fat and losing weight, as well as "Fruits
and Vegetables High in Antioxidants" (Appendix B, page 289).

Eat 2–3 servings of whole grains per day. Another important
way to get lean carbs is through whole grains. Yes, on this diet, you
have permission to eat delicious foods such as bread, oatmeal, whole-
wheat pasta, and brown rice. Whole grains are those containing

100 percent of the entire grain kernel, including the bran, germ, and endosperm. Whole grains also contain fiber, vitamins, minerals, and antioxidants. When shopping for whole grains, look for the "100% Whole Grain" stamp on products. Refined grains, on the other hand, go through a process to remove the bran and germ. The refining process also removes fiber and nutrients.

Carbohydrates have been vilified in the past, but whole grains are an essential part of a healthy diet. That's why the American Heart Association, the 2010 Dietary Guidelines for Americans, the new MyPlate eating guidelines, the Academy of Nutrition and Dietetics (formerly the American Dietetic Association), the Mayo Clinic, the Harvard School of Public Health, and dozens more of the nation's most respected health organizations advocate eating whole grains. Decades of scientific evidence have shown that doing so has been associated with a number of health benefits, which include:

- Reducing the risk of heart disease by 25–28 percent
- Reducing the risk of diabetes by 21–30 percent
- Reducing the risk of stroke by 30–36 percent
- Reducing the risk for metabolic syndrome
- Reducing insulin levels and insulin resistance
- Reducing blood glucose levels
- Reducing total cholesterol
- Reducing LDL cholesterol
- Raising HDL cholesterol
- Reducing triglycerides
- Reducing C-reactive protein, an inflammation marker
- Reducing the risk of inflammatory disease
- Promoting healthier arteries
- Lowering the risk of colorectal cancer
- Reducing blood pressure levels
- Reducing the risk of asthma
- Promoting healthier gums and teeth

Add to this list of remarkable health benefits the fact that a diet rich in whole grains contributes to weight loss. Between 2004 and

2009 alone, there were at least ten studies showing that whole grains promote weight loss, reduce BMI, and in particular, reduce waist circumference. Combine all these benefits, and it's easy to see that whole grains make a whole lot of sense for healthy weight loss.

But how does eating whole-grain bread, cereal, rice, pasta, and more help you get slim and stay slim? For one thing, whole grains are jam-packed with fiber to promote satiety and tone down the hunger

---

Get the Skinny on the Science

Eat Whole Grains to Whittle Your Waist Here are just a few of the many highlights from research showing the relationship between whole grains and weight loss.

A team of researchers from Penn State put two groups of people on the same diet, which included five daily servings of fruits and vegetables, three servings of low-fat dairy products, two servings of lean protein, and four to seven servings of grains depending on their individual calorie needs. The only difference in the diet? One group ate only whole grains while the other group ate refined grains. After twelve weeks, both groups lost an average of 8 to 11 pounds, but the group eating whole grains lost significantly more abdominal fat. Wouldn't you like a trimmer waist so you can wear a smaller pants size?

In the *American Journal College of Nutrition,* researchers investigated the relationship between BMI and whole-grain consumption in women. They found that women who consumed at least one serving of whole grains per day had a significantly lower BMI and waist measurement than women who consumed no whole grains.

In a study of 159 college students appearing in the *Journal of Nutrition and Education Behavior,* researchers found that whole grain intake was highest among students with a healthy weight and lower among those who were overweight or obese.

When researchers from the Netherlands analyzed whole-grain consumption among 4,237 middle-aged adults, they reported in the *European Journal of Nutrition* that for each additional gram of whole-grain consumption in both men and women, the risk of being obese was lower.

hormone ghrelin. A study in the *European Journal of Endocrinology* showed eating a diet high in fiber helps balance ghrelin levels in people carrying around extra pounds. That spells hunger relief.

6-Day Fuel Up Whole-Grain Serving Sizes

If you think a serving of whole-grain cereal is whatever fits into the giant bowl you took out of the cupboard, think again. In our society, we often overestimate serving sizes, and this is one of the problems leading to overeating and weight gain. So what constitutes a serving size? Check out the following list for accurate serving sizes:

- ½ 100% whole-wheat bagel (Lender's or Sara Lee–size frozen bagels, not Iggy's or Dunkin' Donuts size)
- 1 slice 100% whole-wheat bread (1 serving = 1 ounce)
- ½ cup oatmeal, cooked (or ¼ cup dry), old-fashioned or steel cut
- ½ cup Cream of Wheat, cooked (or ¼ cup dry)
- ½ cup oat bran cereal, cooked (or ¼ cup dry)
- 1 serving ready-to-eat, high-fiber cereal (1 serving per nutrition label)
- ⅓ cup brown rice, cooked (or ⅛ cup dry)
- ½ cup whole-wheat pasta, cooked (or 1 ounce dry)
- ½ cup couscous, cooked (or ⅛ cup dry)
- ½ cup quinoa, cooked (or ⅛ cup dry)
- ½ cup farro, cooked (or ¼ cup dry)
- 2 whole-grain crackers (I like Wasa Crisp Bread Crackers)

Prescription 3: Focus on healthy fats, and limit added fats to 4 servings per day.

Just as not all carbohydrates are created equal, neither are all fats. In the United States, we consume too many fatty foods: We eat 110 percent of the recommended amount of saturated fats. This is bad news for our waistlines and for our health. For decades, saturated fats have been associated with increased risk for cardiovascular disease. A seminal study published in the *New England Journal of Medicine* reported that each increase of 5 percent of calories from saturated fat as compared with equivalent intake from carbohydrates was associated with a 17 percent increase in risk of heart disease. Pretty scary stuff, but the questions doctors everywhere were asking was, "What do we use to replace the saturated fat?"

Most of the low-fat diets designed in response to these findings allowed free rein to chow down on carbohydrates in place of those nasty saturated fats, but did not differentiate between whole-grain and refined carbs. But as you now know, eating too many refined carbohydrates has *also* been found to increase the risk for heart disease and diabetes. In fact, they may be even more detrimental to your health than saturated fats. That makes things a little confusing, doesn't it?

Physicians, scientists, and researchers went back to the drawing board and headed back to their labs to do more research. And there have been some important revelations. The message about ditching refined carbohydrates in favor of lean carbs as the Overnight Diet recommends is coming through crystal clear. But what about those fats? Do all types of fat contribute to disease? Or are saturated fats the only villains? Do all fats go immediately to your thighs and belly? Do you have to eliminate all fats if you want to burn fat?

The exciting news is that we are learning that while overeating saturated fats promotes disease and weight gain, eating certain types of fats *in the right amounts* might actually help you burn fat and promote better health. What are these potential fat-burning, disease-fighting fats?

Say hello to PUFAs and MUFAs.

PUFAs are polyunsaturated fatty acids. Unlike saturated fats, which are solid at room temperature, PUFAs are typically in liquid form whether at room temperature or chilled. PUFAs contain essential fatty acids (EFAs) called omega-3 fatty acids and omega-6 fatty acids. Your body needs these for optimal health, but it does not produce enough of them, so you must obtain them from food. Foods you will be eating on the 6-Day Fuel Up that are high in PUFAs include cod, halibut, salmon, shrimp, tuna, tempeh, and tofu. Be aware that not all PUFAs are created equal. Vegetable oils, such as corn, safflower, soybean, and sunflower oil, are high in PUFAs but aren't recommended on the Overnight Diet. That's because when heated, they are easily oxidized, which may have a negative impact on health. You are encouraged to stick to the added fats and fat-free alternatives listed on page 81.

MUFAs are monounsaturated fatty acids. At room temperature, they are typically in liquid form, but when refrigerated, they become solid. These fats are high in vitamin E, an antioxidant. Foods you will be eating on the 6-Day Fuel Up that are high in MUFAs include avocados, nuts, peanut butter, seeds, and olive oil.

If saturated fats are the sticky, gooey stuff that clogs arteries, PUFAs and MUFAs just may be the Liquid-Plumr that unclogs your arteries so your blood can flow more freely. Swapping out saturated fats for PUFAs and MUFAs results in favorable changes in cholesterol levels that boost protection for your heart.

Get the Skinny on the Science

PUFA Power A growing body of research has shown that replacing saturated fats with PUFAs decreases the risk for heart disease. Replacing just 1 percent of saturated fat with PUFAs reduces LDL levels and reduces the risk of coronary events by about 2 to 3 percent, according to a 2011 study in the *American Journal of Clinical Nutrition*. In other research, a team of scientists analyzed the findings from numerous studies on fat and cardiovascular disease and published their review in the *American Journal of Clinical Nutrition*. They found that for every 5 percent reduction in intake from saturated fats that was replaced by a concomitant increase in consumption of PUFAs, there was a 10 percent reduction in the risk for heart disease.

So what about the weight loss aspect? PUFAs and MUFAs have both been shown to enhance weight loss and decrease the inflammation that has been associated with increased abdominal fat and muscle wasting. MUFA consumption has been linked specifically to reduced abdominal fat. One of the most intriguing studies on MUFAs and body fat appeared in *Diabetes Care* and found that premenopausal women who ate more MUFAs maintained more lean muscle mass than women on a very low-fat diet. In other research from the Czech Republic, obese women lost more weight when consuming more PUFAs.

Just because PUFAs and MUFAs are a better choice than saturated fats, it is still important to remember that all fats are highly caloric. All fats—saturated, PUFA, MUFA—provide 9 calories per gram, and they don't rate high in terms of satiety. In fact, research from a 2010 issue of *Nutrition Journal* revealed that there is no difference in satiety whether you eat saturated fats, PUFAs, or MUFAs. Eating PUFAs and MUFAs in the right amount is key. Stick with the portion suggestions in the meal plans and recipes in Chapters 7 and 8 and see the recommendations for added fats below.

Beware of the Trans Fats

One type of fat that can have disastrous effects on your weight and health is trans fats. These fats are used to fry foods like French fries and doughnuts and to help foods like crackers and potato chips have a longer shelf life. They are also found in margarine. On nutrition labels, you can find them listed as "partially hydrogenated vegetable oil." Surprisingly, "fully (or "completely") hydrogenated vegetable oil" does not produce trans fats. Not only do trans fats lead to overall weight gain, but they contribute specifically to abdominal fat, even

---

Get the Skinny on the Science

Trans Fats Transfer Fat to the Belly Researchers at Wake Forest University School of Medicine fed two groups of monkeys a diet that was equal in calories but different in the type of fat consumed. One set of monkeys ate trans fats; the other group ate MUFAs. The number of calories consumed should have maintained their weight without increasing it. But that isn't what happened. The monkeys that ate the trans fats gained 7.2 percent in body weight compared to a 1.8 percent in the monkeys that ate MUFAs. But what was really troublesome was that the extra fat on the monkeys that ate trans fats all settled in the abdomen. Not only that, fat from other areas of the body migrated to the belly.

if you are on a low-calorie diet. Trying to stave off hunger by eating foods like fat-free crackers, cakes, and cookies that are high in trans fats can prevent you from losing the muffin top. Trans fats also raise LDL cholesterol and lower the protective HDL cholesterol, effectively raising the risk for heart disease. There is no place on the Overnight Diet for trans fats. Ditch 'em!

Added Fats. On the Overnight Diet, you don't have to eliminate added fats, but you will be limiting them to up to 4 servings per day (1 serving = 1 teaspoon). Focus on healthy added fats that are high in PUFAs and MUFAs, and understand that there are many ways to add flavor to dishes without adding fat. Simple ways to do so include using cooking sprays made from olive oil, fat-free mayonnaise, and fat-free salad dressings. Just these simple switches can dramatically lower your fat consumption and speed you to faster weight loss.

Added Fat (up to 4 servings/day) (1 serving = 1 teaspoon)	Avocados Low-fat salad dressings Low-fat dips and sauces Mayonnaise (made with olive oil) Non-trans-fat buttery spreads (I like Earth Balance) Olive oil Nuts Seeds
Fat-Free Alternatives	Cooking sprays (made with olive oil) Fat-free dips and sauces Fat-free salad dressings Fat-free mayonnaise

Prescription 4: Drink at least 8 cups of water a day, and feel free to enjoy a glass of wine—just one, however!

Staying adequately hydrated while dieting is absolutely essential to keep fat burning in the fast lane. Here are just a couple of the ways being even slightly dehydrated can cause fat burning to sputter:

- **Dehydration disrupts the metabolism process.** Burning calories creates toxins that need to be flushed out of your body. Your kidneys are your body's chief toxin flushers, and they need water to do their job properly. Dehydration reduces their on-the-job performance, creating a backup of toxins in the body. To prevent a potentially dangerous overload of toxins, your kidneys have to call in the liver for backup. But asking your liver to fill in on toxin-flushing duty takes it away from one of its primary functions: metabolizing fat. Feed your kidneys water so your liver can do its job.

- **Dehydration robs the body of muscle.** Water makes up over 75 percent of your muscles, and it is critical to the process of building lean muscle. It is also essential for reducing muscle cramps and joint pain, both of which can keep you from doing the physical activities that build lean muscle and boost metabolism. Plus, dehydration reduces blood volume, which lowers the supply of oxygen to your muscles and makes them feel tired. Because maintaining lean muscle is at the foundation of rapid fat burning on this diet, you must keep your muscles adequately hydrated. Hydrated muscle cells are stronger and less likely to be gobbled up for energy.

MYTHBUSTERS

MYTH: Drinking water will make you retain water and look bloated. In fact, it's just the opposite. Water retention and the subsequent bloating are signs of *dehydration*. When your body is deprived of adequate water supplies, it sends off a "9-1-1" alert to the brain, which responds by signaling the body's cells to conserve water. It's almost as if your body starts building internal dams to keep any water from escaping, and unfortunately, the biggest reservoir of water usually winds up on your abdomen. If you experience abdominal bloating, it could be a sign that you need to drink more fluids.

For adequate hydration, drink at least eight 8-ounce glasses for a total of 64 ounces, or 2 quarts, of water every day. It doesn't matter if you drink tap water, spring water, seltzer water, or soda water. You can also have flavored waters, as long as they are unsweetened.

On the Overnight Diet, you can also enjoy black coffee, tea, and diet soda (less than 2 calories), but these do not count toward your daily requirement of 64 ounces of water. In fact, caffeinated beverages are *dehydrating.* So if you drink 8 ounces of a caffeinated beverage, you need to offset that by drinking 8 ounces of water—and that's in addition to the 64 ounces.

Get the Skinny on the Science

Drink Before You Eat To lose weight even faster, drink water before your meals. Research presented at the 2010 National Meeting of the American Chemical Society in Boston found that drinking just two cups of water right before you eat increases weight loss. In a trial involving 48 middle-aged and older adults, those who drank water prior to eating consumed an average of 75 to 90 calories fewer at that meal. The researchers suggest that the water made them feel fuller and less hungry. After twelve weeks, the water drinkers lost more weight compared to those who didn't have water before meals, and they kept the weight off for more than a year. In addition, according to German researchers reporting in the *Journal of Clinical Endocrinology and Metabolism*, within ten minutes of drinking 17 ounces of water, metabolic rates in both men and women begin to rise, and they increase by 30 percent after 30 to 40 minutes.

What About Alcohol?

Research shows that having one alcoholic beverage per day offers health benefits. Wine, as opposed to beer or hard liquor, gets the stamp of approval on this diet thanks to the many health benefits associated with moderate wine consumption, including:

- Reduced risk of heart disease
- Increased HDL cholesterol
- Reduced risk of type 2 diabetes
- Reduced risk of cancer
- Reduced risk of stroke
- Slowed progression of neurological degenerative disorders such as Alzheimer's disease
- Reduced cellular damage from free radicals
- Reduced risk of cataracts

You may have heard that red wine is better than white wine when it comes to heart health, but this may not be true. Both red and white wines have been found to offer protection for your heart. Some research shows that a single glass of wine per day can raise levels of HDL cholesterol, the "good" cholesterol. So raise a nightly glass of Chardonnay, Cabernet Sauvignon, or Pinot Noir—absolutely guilt-free. If you don't drink, don't start. If you do, switch to wine.

Tales of the Measuring Tape

"I've been on lots of diets before that had tiny lists of approved foods. I would get so bored eating the same things over and over, I would have to cheat and go on a binge. Now I get to eat so many of my favorite foods, and I get to drink wine! I never feel like I have to cheat. This is a diet I can live with for the rest of my life."

—Jane, 29, dropped 31 pounds and 6 inches off her waist

Putting It All Together

On the Overnight Diet, you'll be using these four prescriptions to create delicious, satisfying meals and snacks. Keeping them in mind, here is an example of what you can eat each day.

___ **minimum ounces protein, adjust to your DPR**	Lean beef, lean pork, poultry, fish, eggs, soy products, meat alternatives, protein powder
Fruits	All you can eat
Nonstarchy vegetables	All you can eat
2 servings dairy (1 serving = 1 cup)	Fat-free or low-fat (1%) yogurt, milk, cottage cheese, cheese, dairy alternatives
2–3 servings whole grains (See serving on page 77)	Bagel, bread, oatmeal, cream of wheat, oat bran, high-protein high-fiber cereal, brown rice, pasta, crackers, quinoa, couscous, farro
Up to 1 serving starchy veggies/legumes (1 serving = 1 cup)	Corn, potatoes, pumpkin, sweet potato, winter squash, yams, yucca, black beans, black-eyed peas, cannellini, chickpeas, kidney beans, lentils, lima beans, navy beans, pinto beans, peas, red beans, split peas, white beans
Up to 4 servings added fats (1 serving = 1 teaspoon)	Avocado, olive oil, low-fat salad dressings, low-fat mayonnaise, low-fat dips and sauces, non–trans fats, buttery spreads, nuts, seeds
Desserts (optional) (1 serving = as described in recipes)	See Chapter 6 for menus and Chapter 8 for recipes
Wine (optional) (1 glass = 6 ounces)	All varieties

Of course, you can get as creative as you'd like. As you'll see in Chapter 6, "28-Day Meal Plan," and Chapter 8, "6-Day Fuel Up Recipes," the options are endless.

CHAPTER 5

Quickie Rev Up

Did you know that logging endless hours on the treadmill while drastically cutting calories could actually be sabotaging your efforts to lose weight? In addition to making you feel starved and exhausted, it won't help you reach your weight goal. What's the problem? The problem is that this combo of eating less and doing more cardio can put the body into a catabolic state in which it robs the muscles for fuel, effectively slowing metabolism and disrupting the fat-burning process. What should you be doing instead?

As you have already seen, maintaining or developing lean muscle mass is the key to rapid weight loss that lasts and avoiding the Shrinking Muscle Syndrome, so your workout needs to focus on increasing lean muscle. But this doesn't mean you have to follow some run-of-the-mill weight-lifting routine. Recent research has revealed that integrating two exercise concepts into one—similar to the way the Overnight Diet combines two diets into one—burns more fat faster than any other workout. It's like getting twice the results in half the time.

This workout plan relies on a growing body of research showing that combining resistance training with short cardio blasts, called "Rev Up Blasts" here, into one workout can burn almost ten times more body fat compared to doing strength training and cardio separately. This dynamic approach allows you to strengthen and resculpt your body quickly. The moves are designed specifically to help you tackle those trouble spots, including your tummy, butt, thighs, and

---

Get the Skinny on the Science

Reprogram Your DNA If you've logged way too much time on the couch, you might think it's too late for exercise to do your body any good. You'd be wrong! Research in a 2012 issue of *Cell Metabolism* shows that when inactive but otherwise healthy men and women exercise—even for just a few minutes—it results in immediate changes in their DNA. The DNA molecules within the muscles undergo chemical and structural changes that appear to reprogram the muscles for strength and the metabolic benefits of exercise. This is strong evidence that it is never too late to start exercising and, more important, feel the benefits of exercise.

---

jiggly arms. And you can get started today, regardless of your age or fitness level. Even better, you don't have to lift a single barbell or pound away on the treadmill.

Two studies in the *Journal of Strength and Conditioning* tested the effectiveness of a traditional workout versus an integrated workout. Here are the two programs the women participating in the study followed 3 days a week for 11 weeks:

Group 1—Traditional Workout	Group 2—Integrated Workout
Warm-up	Warm-up
Resistance exercises	Alternate between:
Aerobics	high-intensity cardio blast
Cool down	and resistance exercises
	Cool down

The integrated workout produced greater gains in lean muscle, strength, endurance, flexibility, and fat-free mass. It also produced a markedly greater decline in fat mass and reduction in body fat percentage. In fact, it produced an almost tenfold greater reduction in body fat compared to the group doing the traditional workout.

The Quickie Rev Up Burns Fat Faster

Let's take a look at how this workout will kick fat burning into high gear.

Increases metabolism. This workout program increases lean muscle, and the more lean muscle tissue you have, the higher your basic metabolic rate will be. As you've already seen, a higher metabolism pumps up your body's fat-burning potential throughout the day. Muscle burns seven times more calories than fat. This means that the more lean muscle you have, the more efficient your body will be at burning calories. Classic research from Tufts University and the University of Maryland found that strength training increases basic metabolic rate by 7 percent and boosts daily calorie expenditure by 15 percent.

Tales of the Measuring Tape

"I have two toddlers and definitely don't have time to spend an hour a day working out. I needed something that would give me results in a short amount of time. The Quickie Rev Up is the solution. I look more toned than ever, and I love it. I'm wearing tank tops again!"

—Kristen, 32, lost 21 pounds

Ramps up the "after burn." When you alternate between cardio bursts and resistance training moves, you increase something known in scientific circles as excess post-exercise oxygen consumption (EPOC), but which we'll refer to here as the "after burn." Basically, the after burn is the number of calories you burn as your body recovers from a workout and returns to a resting state. This means that after you have finished your workout, your body will continue to burn more calories, even while you are watching TV, reading a book, or sleeping.

Reduces appetite and food cravings. Research shows that strength training can have an almost instantaneous as well as a long-term effect on appetite and those pesky food cravings that threaten to sabotage your weight loss. For several hours following a strength training session, appetite and cravings decrease. In the long run, building lean muscle through strength training has been found to help balance the appetite hormones, which are often out of whack in overweight and obese people. Cardio alone, on the other hand, does not kill appetite, according to Jim Karas, author of the *New York Times* bestseller *The Cardio-Free Diet.*

Burns more belly fat. Interval training, which is similar to the Rev Up cardio blasts you will be doing with the Quickie Rev Up, targets belly fat. It involves alternating between brief bouts of high-intensity activity with periods of lower-intensity exercise, which is exactly what this program is designed to do. In fact, a team of Australian researchers showed that obese women who did interval training lost three times as much body fat—and significantly more fat from their waistlines—than obese women who performed exercise at a continuous pace.

Reduces insulin resistance. As you saw in Chapter 2, the Shrinking Muscle Syndrome is associated with insulin resistance, which is

Get the Skinny on the Science

Research has shown that the components of this workout enhance insulin sensitivity. For example, a report in the *International Journal of Medical Sciences* found that resistance training improves muscle quality and insulin sensitivity in people with type 2 diabetes. In this study, researchers at the University of Maryland tested insulin levels, fat-free mass, body fat percentage, and strength in men ages fifty to sixty-three both before and after 16 weeks of strength training. At the end of the trial, the men's insulin levels had decreased significantly, signaling an improvement in insulin sensitivity. The drop in insulin was accompanied by a 47 percent increase in overall strength, a rise in lean tissue, and a decrease in body-fat percentage. Other research from 2006 in *The Journal of Clinical Endocrinology and Metabolism* also reported that strength training increased insulin sensitivity in obese men.

a contributing factor in water retention and bloating, both of which make you more likely to have extra padding around your midsection. This workout was formulated specifically to help prevent or reverse the Shrinking Muscle Syndrome and the insulin resistance that comes with it. The more lean muscle you have, the more effectively your body uses insulin, thereby reducing insulin resistance so you can eliminate water retention and bloating.

Interval training has also been found to enhance insulin sensitivity. In one study from 2009 in *BMC Endocrine*, just two weeks of interval training produced a 23 percent increase in insulin sensitivity.

Boosts generation of mitochondria. Mitochondria, as discussed, are the small powerhouses within your cells that burn food for energy. Evidence shows that exercise causes an upsurge in the numbers of new mitochondria within the cells of your muscles, which enhances muscle vitality, reduces fatigue, and improves endurance. Even more exciting is the fact that an uptick in mitochondria reduces the risk for obesity and diabetes. Some research shows that the more muscle groups involved in the exercise you do, the higher the increase in mitochondria. With this exercise program, you'll be engaging nearly every muscle group in your body.

Increases levels of HGH. As you have seen, higher levels of HGH are associated with increases in lean muscle mass and reductions in body fat. The two elements of this hybrid workout have been found to be the ideal combo to naturally boost production of the hormone that has been proven to reduce body fat and increase lean muscle mass. Research in *Mechanisms of Ageing and Development* found that strength training can induce the release of HGH in both the young and the elderly, with a greater amount seen in younger people. In 2000, the *Journal of Strength and Conditioning* reported a boost in HGH levels in women following a strength training session, and it didn't matter if the women regularly engaged in strength training or were novices.

The release of HGH following strength training comes as part of the muscle breakdown and regeneration cycle mentioned earlier.

As you learned, adequate protein intake is essential to avoid getting stuck in breakdown mode. So is HGH. Strength training causes tiny tears in the muscles and stimulates production of HGH, which is involved in repairing the muscles.

As a reminder, *the Overnight Diet does not suggest that you take HGH supplements to help you achieve your weight-loss goals.*

Increases energy levels. Physical activity boosts production of AMP kinase, a metabolic enzyme that provides cellular energy, which puts a little more pep in your step and gives you the energy you need to get off the couch and move more. AMP kinase gives you more energy throughout the day and minimizes fatigue. Research shows that AMP kinase is lower in obese people who are insulin resistant compared to obese people who are insulin sensitive.

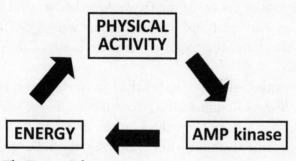

The Energy Solution

Balances your appetite hormones and fights visceral fat with better sleep. Regular exercise has long been associated with improved sleep. In addition to improving your mood during the day, this perk is also something that could be far more beneficial to weight loss than you ever realized. In 2011, the *American Journal of Clinical Nutrition* published a report showing that when you skimp on sleep, you end up eating more. The study involved fifteen men and fifteen women who slept, in random order, for nine hours a night for five nights and four hours a night for five nights. After getting just four hours of shut-eye for five nights, the study volunteers ate an average of nearly 300 calories more than when they slept for nine hours a night. And those calories came mostly from fat and most notably saturated fat.

Research shows that sleep deprivation wreaks havoc with the body's appetite hormones and leads to visceral fat, the dangerous fat that wraps around your vital organs. In 2010, the National Sleep Foundation reported a 32 percent increase in visceral fat in people under the age of forty who slept less than six hours a night.

Other research shows that a shortage of sleep causes a decrease in leptin, the satiety hormone that signals the brain that the body is full, and an increase in ghrelin, the hormone that triggers hunger. The end result? No matter how much you eat, you feel hungry, which makes you more likely to overeat. Getting adequate shut-eye—at least six hours per night—helps balance the appetite hormones, which are primarily produced at night, so it will be easier to control your appetite during the waking hours. And don't think that you can just "catch up" on sleep on the weekends. To maintain these benefits, you need to get six or more hours of sleep on a consistent basis.

Increases the release of adrenaline to burn stored fat. According to Dr. Steven Boutcher, the Australian professor who has done groundbreaking research on the kind of short cardio blasts you'll be doing on this workout, they pump up the release of the hormone adrenaline. That's a good thing for weight loss because adrenaline plays a role in breaking down stored fat and burning it. Adrenaline also dampens the appetite, so you'll feel less hungry *while* you're burning more fat.

Reduces levels of the stress hormone that makes you fat. Everybody knows that when you feel stressed, you tend to reach for foods that make you fat—chocolate chip cookies, cheeseburgers, or chips, for example. It's no surprise that people who experience a lot of pressure tend to pack on the pounds. Research shows us that stress and fat feed off each other. When you're under chronic strain, your body releases too much of the stress hormone cortisol, and too much cortisol is what can make you crave and overeat high-fat junk foods. People who are overweight or obese tend to have high levels of cortisol, but so do people who have excess abdominal fat but are slim otherwise. And who wants to have slender arms and legs but a bulging belly? When you exercise on a regular basis, it not only decreases stress, but it also improves your resilience in handling high-pressure situations. And it reduces cortisol levels, which can help you win the battle against stress eating and stress-related weight gain.

Improves your mood to reduce overeating. The mood-boosting benefits of exercise have been well documented, and the proof keeps rolling in. For example, a 2012 study from researchers at Penn State shows that people who get more physical activity tend to feel more excitement and enthusiasm compared to people who are less physically active. These positive feelings may in part be due to the fact that exercise enhances the production of the body's natural feel-good neurochemical endorphin, providing an almost instantaneous mood boost. Not only is this great for your mood, but it is also amazing for your waistline. These endorphins also act as an appetite suppressant to help keep eating under control.

Physical activity has also been found to soothe anxiety, relieve blue moods, and even reduce the incidence of clinical depression, all of which may be triggers for emotional overeating. One in ten U.S. adults suffers from depression, according to the Centers for Disease Control, and unfortunately these people are more likely to be obese, too. A growing body of research points to a link between depression and obesity. The good news? A 2011 review of the scientific evidence on the effect of physical activity on mild depression has found that exercise and physical activity are as effective as antidepressant treatments.

Reduces the risk of injury so you can stay active. When you place stress on your bones through activity, such as strength training, your body responds by reinforcing those bones in a process similar to the breakdown and regeneration of muscle that also occurs with strength training. Having stronger bones makes you less likely to develop osteoporosis or experience bone fractures that can keep you off your feet. Toning your muscles also strengthens the ligaments and tendons that support your joints, reducing your chance of injuries such as sprains and strains. When you are injury-free, you are more likely to remain active throughout your lifetime!

Improves immune system function. Nothing slows you down like a nasty cold or flu bug. A wealth of scientific research proves that regular exercise shores up your immune system so you can fight off viruses and infections that might derail your efforts to stay active.

Reduces the risk for chronic disease. Decades of research show that regular exercise reduces your risk for heart disease, stroke, cancer, high blood pressure, diabetes, and other debilitating diseases. Regular physical activity strengthens the heart muscle, increases the protective HDL cholesterol, reduces the harmful LDL cholesterol, improves blood flow, reduces blood pressure, improves insulin sensitivity, and more. When you aren't sidelined by disease, you are more inclined to remain active.

Why You'll Love This Workout

Fast fat burning isn't the only benefit you'll enjoy from the Quickie Rev Up. This fun, fast-paced workout strengthens nearly every major muscle group in the body while improving balance and flexibility at the same time. Fun and functional for everyday life, these moves will help you do the things you love to do—chase after your toddler at the park, take your dog for a hike, or play a round of golf—*and* do them better and more effortlessly! How would you like to hustle up the stairs without huffing and puffing? Play tennis without needing to down a whole bottle of Advil afterward? Or go dancing without feeling like you're going to throw your back out?

Of course, you want all the benefits that come with regular exercise, but you're busy and don't have hours to dedicate to a workout routine. That's why the Quickie Rev Up has been engineered to provide maximum results in the least amount of time possible. All it takes is 21 minutes four times a week. Out of a total of 10,080 minutes in each week, this routine takes up only 84 of them. Just 84 out of 10,080—that's less than 1 percent of your week! It's a routine that can fit into the craziest hustle-and-bustle lifestyle.

> ## Tales of the Measuring Tape
>
> *"I was always afraid that strength training would make me look big and bulky. Boy, was I wrong! I'm leaner than ever, and my body looks toned but totally feminine. For the first time in my life, I feel confident enough to wear a bikini."*　　　—Caroline, 31, lost 37 pounds

The Quickie Rev Up won't leave you yawning from boredom either. With ten different strength-training moves to choose from and ten different ways to do the Rev Up Blasts, this routine keeps you and your muscles guessing to prevent the fitness plateaus that occur when doing the same exercises over and over. After all, your body is incredibly smart. It adapts quickly to exercise, becoming so efficient at the various moves that it takes less and less effort to perform them.

When you first start the program, you may find some of the moves very challenging. But after just a few weeks, your body will adapt to these moves and you will find that they seem easier and that you are ready to pump up intensity. This is progress! But your body is so good at adapting that if you do the same moves over and over and over, you may stop seeing that progress. To avoid such plateaus, you need to switch up your workout routine. Changing up a couple of the moves you do or doing them in a different order may be all it takes to keep challenging your muscles so you keep getting leaner and more toned.

> ## Tales of the Measuring Tape
>
> *"I thought I was too fat to exercise, but the Quickie Rev Up offered ways to make each of the moves easier. So I just did the easier options at first and that gave me the confidence I needed to keep going. Now I'm doing the more advanced options, which I never would have imagined I could do. I look and feel like a completely different person."*　　　—Alberto, 51, lost 109 pounds

Rest assured, this workout can be tailored for all fitness levels. If you're a complete novice, you don't need to feel intimidated because the moves can be modified to make them easier. And you can rev up the intensity as you progress.

One of the best things about the Quickie Rev Up is that it requires almost nothing besides your body. You don't have to join a fancy, expensive gym or invest in a bunch of pricey equipment. You can do it anytime, anywhere—in your own home, at a park, or in a hotel room if you're on the road. Of course, if you enjoy working out with weights or like the idea of going to a gym, you'll see how to do the exercises with weights or machines, too. The choice is up to you. Illustrations will show you exactly how to do each move.

MYTHBUSTERS

MYTH: Strength training makes women bulk up and look manly.
If you're afraid that strength training is going to make you look like the Incredible Hulk, stop your fretting. Rest assured, the Quickie Rev Up is not designed to make you bulk up like a hard-core bodybuilder. It's designed first and foremost to help you *maintain* the muscle you already have so you can avoid the Shrinking Muscle Syndrome. Any increases in lean tissue will simply give you a fitter, more toned appearance. Bulking up typically results from a combination of several contributing factors, including lifting heavy weights (which you won't be doing), dedicating several hours a day to weight training (which you won't be doing), the hormone testosterone (which women do not produce in sufficient quantities to increase muscle size), and a caloric surplus (which you won't have on this diet).

Check with your physician before starting any exercise program.

Quickie Rev Up Basics

The workout starts with a Dynamic Warm Up then alternates between strength training moves and 60-second Rev Up Blasts. It is most important to keep it quick! It is called the Quickie Rev Up for three reasons. First, the whole thing takes just 21 minutes. Second, it is engineered to reshape your body quickly. And third, it is important that you go from move to move quickly without taking any breaks. As soon as you complete the Dynamic Warm Up, jump right into your first strength-training move then hustle into your first Rev Up Blast and back to the next strength training move. It'll be over before you know it. Now let's break it down.

Dynamic Warm Up. Forget about the static stretching your high school gym teacher might have had you do to "warm up" before gym class. Emerging research shows that this type of old-school stretching actually reduces performance and may even increase the risk of injury, while a Dynamic Warm Up boosts your athletic abilities and helps prevent sprains and muscle strains. In fact, according to Australian researcher James Zois at the School of Sport and Exercise Science at Victoria University in Melbourne, there is an 11 percent difference in performance depending on whether you do static stretching or a Dynamic Warm Up before physical activity—with the Dynamic Warm Up coming out on top.

This do-anywhere first step prepares your body to crank up your performance for even faster results while minimizing the risk for injury. It consists of five simple moves that you will do in rapid succession for a total of 3 minutes, but we'll get into the specifics in Chapter 9. In just those 3 minutes, this warm up will:

- Activate your muscles from head to toe.
- Warm up your muscles and ligaments to prevent injury.
- Open up your joints to improve mobility.
- Wake up your nervous system to help your body coordinate your movement.
- Increase blood flow to send more oxygen to the muscles.

The Dynamic Warm Up is essential in helping you get the most out of the Quickie Rev Up, *so don't skip it.*

Strength Training Moves. As we've discussed, strength training is absolutely essential for maintaining lean muscle mass and preventing the Shrinking Muscle Syndrome. Starting at age twenty-five, adults who don't strength train lose an average of at least half a pound of lean muscle tissue each year. And only 21 percent of women strength train two or more times per week, according to the National Center for Health Statistics. This means that four out of five women are losing lean muscle tissue right now. It is estimated that people lose 30 percent of their muscle strength between the ages of fifty and seventy.

The only way to develop lean muscle mass is to expose the muscles to some form of resistance, such as your own body weight, free weights, or machines. During strength training, which may also be referred to as resistance training, muscle fibers are broken down and then quickly repaired by the body. Remember when we discussed your body being like a factory? After strength training, your factory workers rush in to mend the torn or injured muscle fibers, and they throw in some extra padding (aka more fibers) while they're at it to help shore up those muscles. It is this ongoing cycle of breakdown and repair that preserves and builds lean muscle.

Most people are surprised to discover that it isn't the strength training that actually makes muscles get bigger. Rather, it's the repair process that is set in motion to heal the tiny "injuries" to the muscles caused by resistance training that ultimately strengthens them and increases their size. The repair process starts taking place almost immediately after you complete a resistance-training workout.

The body weight moves here are designed to provide the resistance you need to break down muscle tissue and stimulate the repair process. They incorporate several muscle groups at once so you get more results in less time. There are five Quickie Rev Up Foundation Moves and five Quickie Rev Up Advanced Moves. They are called Foundation Moves because they provide the foundation for the more advanced exercises. This is why it is critical that you learn them first. Regardless of your current fitness level, it is recommended that you spend at least two weeks doing the five Foundation Moves before tackling the Advanced Moves. But don't feel pressured to progress to the Advanced Moves. The Foundation Moves work nearly every muscle in your body, so if they continue to provide enough challenge for you week after week, stick with them! Along with the basics of each move, you'll find tips on how to make it easier or how to increase the intensity depending on your fitness level.

In Chapter 9, you will find illustrations and easy-to-follow step-by-step instructions for each of the body-weight moves customized for all fitness levels. You can mix and match with simple routines that alternate in order to continually challenge the muscles, which will prevent them—and you—from getting bored. Even if you are doing the five Quickie Rev Up Foundation Moves, you should change up the order in which you do them to prevent boredom.

MYTHBUSTERS

MYTH: Strength training makes your muscles so sore, you can barely move the next day. If you wake up the morning after doing your Quickie Rev Up routine and feel like you got run over by a truck, you've probably overdone it and should scale back the intensity of your workout. Strength training at the appropriate intensity will likely cause mild muscle soreness the following day, or rather "muscle awareness." This means you are aware of the muscles you worked and you can tell that you challenged them, but they are not achy. If you are very sore, take a day off to rest your muscles before exercising again. If soreness is due to an injury, check with your physician before exercising.

Rev Up Blasts. These cardio blasts will get your heart pumping and fire up fat burning by depleting the glycogen stores in your muscles. They will also boost your cardiovascular endurance and give you that feel-good endorphin rush. And the best part is they only take 60 seconds. You don't have to jog for an hour on the treadmill, spend 45 minutes climbing on the stair climber, or force yourself to do 30 minutes on the elliptical machine. You go as hard as you can for 60 seconds. To get the most bang for your buck from the Rev Up

Blasts, you really have to give it your all. You can do anything for 60 seconds, right?

The Quickie Rev Up provides ten simple ways to do the 60-second Rev Up Blasts, including speed walking and jogging in place. Again these don't require any equipment, so you can do them anywhere, anytime. The most important thing to remember is that it's quickly jumping from the strength-training moves to the Rev Up Blasts and back again that works magic on your muscles and fires up metabolism. Don't skip one or the other. As with the combination of the 1-Day Power Up and the 6-Day Fuel Up, it's the combination of the strength-training moves and Rev Up Blasts that make this workout the fastest fat burner you can find.

Sample Quickie Rev Up Workout	
Dynamic Warm Up	3 minutes
Strength Training Move	2 minutes
Rev Up Blast	1 minute
Strength Training Move	2 minutes
Rev Up Blast	1 minute
Strength Training Move	2 minutes
Rev Up Blast	1 minute
Strength Training Move	2 minutes
Rev Up Blast	1 minute
Strength Training Move	2 minutes
Rev Up Blast	1 minute
Strength Training Move	2 minutes
Rev Up Blast	1 minute

What Should You Eat and Drink Before and After the Quickie Rev Up?

As a general rule, the energy you use during exercise doesn't come from the food you put in your body immediately prior to working out. It's the glycogen stored in your muscles and fat cells that fuel your workout. With the Overnight Diet, you will be filling up on foods that fuel your muscles and boost your energy and you will be staying adequately hydrated. This means you don't need to stress about preworkout snacks.

What about after your workout? That's a different story. As you recall, strength training breaks down muscle tissue. To put a halt to that breakdown process and to fuel the recovery and repair process that rebuilds and grows your muscles, you need protein; protein is the building block of muscle, after all. Ideally, you should eat something that contains lean protein within half an hour of completing the Quickie Rev Up. Doing so will help stimulate the repair process that will give you the long, lean, toned muscles you want. That glycogen in your muscles you just spent on your workout needs to be replaced as well. On the Overnight Diet, fruits and vegetables along with whole grains do the trick. If you don't have time for a full meal, try a protein-filled snack with healthy carbs to promote the repair-and-replenish process. Here are a few good examples:

- Nonfat Greek yogurt with berries
- Plain, nonfat yogurt with a spoonful of protein powder and an apple
- Nonfat cottage cheese with pineapple tidbits
- ½ turkey sandwich on whole-wheat bread
- 1 hard-boiled egg and 1 slice whole-wheat toast

On the days you do the Quickie Rev Up, it is a good idea to drink at least 8 ounces of water prior to starting your workout, another 8 ounces of water while you work out, and 8 ounces more after you finish to aid the recovery process. If you sweat excessively or it is extremely hot or humid, you may need even more fluids.

Quickie Rev Up Fitness Assessment

Whether you have never broken a sweat in your entire life or you are a regular exerciser, the Quickie Rev Up can be tailored to suit your individual needs. It is important to work at the appropriate level to prevent injury and to help you stay motivated so you can get the maximum fat-burning effect. Trying an advanced routine when you are a beginner can be demoralizing and make you want to throw in the towel. But when you work out at the appropriate level for you, you will see progress quickly and be able to enjoy a slimmer, trimmer, more toned body faster than you ever thought possible. Answer the following questions to find your fitness level so you can get the most out of Quickie Rev Up:

1. **What is your age?**
   A. Over 50
   B. 30–49
   C. Under 30

2. **What is your BMI?**
   A. Over 35
   B. 30–35
   C. Under 30

3. **How often are you physically active?**
   A. I don't engage in any physical activity.
   B. I participate in physical activity occasionally (less than three times per week).
   C. I am physically active on a regular basis (at least three times per week).

4. **Do you strength train?**
   A. I have never done strength training.
   B. I have done strength training but do not do it on a regular basis (less than twice a week).
   C. I do strength training regularly (at least twice a week).

5. **Which best describes your ability to do a push-up?**
   A. I can't do any kind of push-up.
   B. I can do at least one push-up with my knees touching the floor.
   C. I can do at least one traditional push-up.

6. How much cardio endurance do you have?

A. I get tired going from the couch to the fridge.

B. I can walk briskly for 5–15 minutes before getting tired.

C. I can walk briskly more than 15 minutes without getting tired.

7. Which best describes your flexibility?

A. I don't even come close to touching my toes when I bend over.

B. When I bend over, my fingertips are within a couple of inches of my toes.

C. I can put my fingertips or whole hands on the floor when I bend over.

8. Do you have any chronic aches or pains (back, knees, hips, feet, etc.)?

A. I am in constant pain.

B. I have some issues with pain but not all the time.

C. I do not have chronic pain.

Mostly A's: Make It Easier

You're new to fitness or it's been a while since you've broken a sweat, and you may have some issues with pain that have kept you on the sidelines. Use the "Make It Easier" options for the five Quickie Rev Up Foundation Moves for at least two weeks or until you get the hang of the exercises and build up your confidence, strength, and endurance. When you feel comfortable with the "Make It Easier" versions, you can step up to the basic versions and pat yourself on the back for a job well done.

Mostly B's: Basic Move

You may be like so many busy people who sporadically squeeze in a workout here and there. Or maybe you are one of those people who go through phases—working out like crazy for a few months and then dropping it altogether. Developing consistency is key to igniting the breakdown and repair processes that increase lean muscle mass to keep fat burning in the fast lane. Start with the "Basic Move" options of the five Quickie Rev Up Foundation Moves for at least two full weeks before advancing to the "Rev It Up" options.

Mostly C's: Rev It Up

You engage in some form of exercise on a regular basis and are probably raring to take advantage of the fat-burning potential of the Quickie Rev Up. Start with the "Rev It Up" versions of the five Quickie Rev Up Foundation Moves for the first two weeks before progressing to the Quickie Rev Up Advanced Moves. It is important that you master the proper form and technique of these moves to see maximum fat-burning results.

PART III

THE OVERNIGHT DIET MADE EASY

28-Day Meal Plan

On most diets, you have to starve yourself into your skinny jeans. Not on this one. When you look at the following 28-day meal plan, you'll be amazed by how much food—and how many *kinds* of food— you get to eat. You'll be enjoying pancakes, pizza, breakfast tacos, chili, burgers, even cheesecake—all while burning fat and dropping pounds. It's time for you to say good-bye to hunger and deprivation and hello to a delicious bounty of satisfying food.

How to Use Chapter 6

The 28-day meal plan offers an easy-to-follow blueprint. The 1-Day Power Up days, which fall on Day 1 of each week, are a cinch— three delicious, satisfying, jumbo smoothies that will torch fat while keeping hunger at bay. On the 6-Day Fuel Up days, you'll be eating breakfast, lunch, and dinner, plus three snacks a day (optional) and dessert (optional). The 6-Day Fuel Up days have been created with the four prescriptions from Chapter 4 in mind:

Prescription 1: Meet your DPR every day.

Prescription 2: Stick to lean carbs. Nosh on a bottomless buffet of fruits and nonstarchy vegetables, eat up to 1 cup of starchy veggies and 2–3 servings of whole grains absolutely guilt-free.

Prescription 3: Focus on healthy fats, but remember there can be too much of a good thing—only eat up to 4 servings daily.

Prescription 4: Drink at least 8 cups of fluids a day, and feel free to enjoy one glass of wine.

Important! Adjust Protein Quantities to Meet Your DPR: The daily meal plans here have been designed for someone with a DPR of 14, which means they provide about 14 ounces of lean protein per day on the 6-Day Fuel Up. Referring back to the chart in Chapter 4, women who have an *ideal* weight of about 140 to 149 pounds and men with an *ideal* weight of about 142 to 153 pounds have a DPR of 14 ounces. Depending on your individual DPR, you will need to adjust the amount of protein in the daily meal plans to meet your needs.

Remember, the protein sources that count toward your DPR for the 6-Day Fuel Up are:

- Lean beef
- Lean pork
- Fish
- Poultry
- Eggs
- Soy products and meat alternatives
- Protein powder

It is imperative that you adjust the quantities of these specific protein sources in this meal plan and in the recipes to meet your individual minimum DPR. To make it easier for you, the recipes in Chapter 8 indicate the protein sources you need to adjust. But note that there is no need to adjust any other ingredients or serving sizes.

Here's how to do it: The meal plan is designed to provide 14 ounces of protein a day: 2 ounces at breakfast, 4 ounces at lunch, and 8 ounces at dinner. When adjusting recipes for your DPR, the simplest thing to do is look at the day's meals that specify protein in ounces—say, 4 ounces of salmon as on Week 1, Day 5, on page 118— and add or subtract what you need. If your DPR is 13 ounces per day, you would *subtract* 1 ounce and have 3 ounces of salmon. If your DPR is 15 ounces, you would *add* an ounce and have 5 ounces. All the other meals on that day would stay the same. That's the only adjustment you would need to make.

But what if the day's plan—like Week 1, Day 2, on page 115—is made up of meals such as Spicy Chicken and White Bean Chili, which yields 4 servings, and Crusty Oven-Fried Fish, which yields 4 servings? Again, it's simple. At the top of each recipe in Chapter 8, you'll see "Protein per Serving Toward DPR," which shows you how many ounces of protein are in each serving. You can either adjust both lunch and dinner to meet your needs or modify only one of those meals and leave the rest of the day's meals the same. Whatever is simplest for you. Remember, it's your daily protein *total* that is most important.

To illustrate this adjustment, let's look at how two different people, both with unique DPRs, would make adjustments for Week 1, Day 5 (4 ounces salmon for lunch) and Week 1, Day 2 (1 serving Spicy Chicken and White Bean Chili for lunch and 1 serving Crusty Oven-Fried Fish for dinner).

- Kim's ideal weight is 110, so her DPR is 12 ounces of protein per day. Remember, 12 ounces is the *minimum* DPR for all adults, regardless of your ideal weight. And since your DPR is the *minimum* amount of protein you should be consuming, Kim isn't *required* to decrease the amount of protein in the daily meal plans. But if she wants to, she can reduce the daily meal plans by 2 ounces of protein per day.
- Mark's ideal weight is 184, so his DPR is 18 ounces of protein per day. He needs to add 4 ounces of protein per day.

Kim, with a DPR of 12 ounces, can reduce the daily meal plans by 2 ounces of protein per day.

Week 1, Day 5: Instead of 4 ounces of salmon at lunch, Kim would have 2 ounces of salmon and the rest of the day's meals would remain the same.

Week 1, Day 2: To eliminate 2 ounces of protein, Kim could reduce lunch and dinner by 1 ounce each or simply reduce dinner by

2 ounces. Here's how. The chili recipe calls for 16 ounces of chicken breast for 4 servings, which means there are 4 ounces of chicken in each serving. Reducing each serving by 1 ounce means she would need 3 ounces of chicken per serving, or a total of 12 ounces to make 4 servings. The fish recipe calls for 4 8-ounce pieces of cod. Simply adjust that to 4 pieces that are 7 ounces each. This way, Kim has eliminated 1 ounce from lunch and 1 ounce from dinner. She could also keep one of the recipes as is, say the chili recipe, and modify only the fish recipe, reducing each serving by 2 ounces so she would use 4 6-ounce pieces of cod. There is no need to alter any other ingredient amounts in the recipes.

Mark, with a DPR of 18 ounces, needs to add 4 ounces of protein per day to daily meal plans.

Week 1, Day 5: Instead of 4 ounces of salmon at lunch, Mark would have 8 ounces of salmon, and the rest of the day's meals would remain the same.

Week 1, Day 2: To add 4 ounces of protein, he could add 2 ounces to each lunch and dinner or simply add 4 ounces to dinner.

Here's how. The chili recipe calls for 16 ounces of chicken breast for 4 servings, which means there are 4 ounces of chicken in each serving. Increasing each serving by 2 ounces means he would need 6 ounces of chicken per serving, or a total of 24 ounces of chicken to make 4 servings. The fish recipe calls for 4 8-ounce pieces of cod. Simply adjust that to 4 pieces that are 10 ounces each. This way, Jim has added 2 ounces to lunch and 2 ounces to dinner. He could also keep one of the recipes as is, say the chili recipe, and modify only the fish recipe, increasing each serving by 4 ounces so he would use 4 12-ounce pieces of cod. There is no need to alter any other ingredient amounts in the recipes.

Converting Grams to Ounces: Because nutrition labels indicate nutrient content in grams, you'll need to convert grams to ounces on the fly while grocery shopping for ingredients. All you have to do to is divide the number of grams by 7 (there are 7 grams of protein to

1 ounce of protein). For example, if something has 28 grams of protein, you divide by 7 and get 4 ounces of protein.

Examples Converting Grams to Ounces of Protein
28 grams protein ÷ 7 = 4 ounces protein
15 grams protein ÷ 7 = 2.1 ounces protein
9 grams protein ÷ 7 = 1.3 ounces protein

Meal Plan Dos and Don'ts

- Do start with the 1-Day Power Up on Day 1 and each week thereafter.
- Do follow the four prescriptions for the 6-Day Fuel Up on Days 2–7 of each week.
- Don't skip any meals (it's okay to skip snacks and dessert; they're optional) or you won't be getting adequate protein.
- Don't combine meals, for example eating lunch and dinner all together in one huge meal. The body can process only so much protein at one time, so the protein-packed meals are best when spread throughout the day.

Take advantage of flexibility. Flexibility is an integral part of this program, so even though smoothies, meals, and snacks are clearly outlined, feel free to make substitutions within the parameters of the diet. For example, the three smoothies listed for Day 1 of each week have been selected to spark weight loss and ensure a variety of flavors. But Chapter 7 will give you more details on how to select three smoothies of your choosing for your 1-Day Power Up. You can also replace one of the suggested smoothies with one of your own creation using the "Mix 'n' Match Smoothie Chart" (Appendix A, page 279). You'll find more on this in Chapter 7, too.

The 6-Day Fuel Up recommendations are also interchangeable. If you don't eat pork, it's okay to have chicken, beef, fish, or soy products instead. If you aren't a fan of broccoli, but you do like spinach, then by all means have spinach. If you prefer brown rice to couscous, go with the whole grain you prefer. Just be sure to make these types of substitutions in equal measures—if the meal plan calls for 1 serving of couscous (½ cup, cooked), then swap it for 1 serving of brown rice (⅓ cup, cooked), and so on. And remember, coffee, tea, in-between meal snacks, dessert, and a nightly glass of wine are all optional.

Meal timing. Meal timing is also flexible. One question that gets asked a lot is: "How long do I wait in between meals and snacks?" Generally, it's a good idea to space out meals and snacks every two to three hours. Here's how this might look:

8 a.m.	Breakfast
10:30 a.m.	Snack
1 p.m.	Lunch
3:30 p.m.	Snack
6 p.m.	Dinner and dessert
8:30 p.m.	Snack

Sticking to this type of schedule is advisable because it helps prevent hunger throughout the day. Of course, with a hectic lifestyle, it is not always possible. You might have a crazy day at work and not get around to eating lunch until 3 o'clock. You might have to shuttle the kids from school to soccer practice to a playdate and miss your afternoon snack. Or you might be a student who keeps funny hours and ends up eating dinner at 11 p.m. That's what happened to Melinda, a patient at the Nutrition and Weight Management Center at Boston Medical Center who was going to medical school. She had classes all day long then spent long hours studying at the library and sometimes wouldn't get around to dinner until late at night. That's okay. Occasionally getting off schedule won't disrupt the metabolic improvements provided by the Overnight Diet. However, if you find that you are regularly off schedule, be sure to keep your bottomless buffet of fruits and veggies on hand for snacking to tide you over until you have a chance to eat your meal.

Grocery shopping guide. Having all the ingredients you need for the week's meals and smoothies on hand helps ensure your weight-loss success. To make sure you're prepared for the coming week, take time on your R&R 1-Day Power Up to review the entire week of menus, make shopping lists (consult "The Overnight Diet Shopping List" in Appendix B, page 283), and hit the market. If you see that some of the week's recipes are best made a day or two in advance, consider preparing them on your R&R day. Look for these and other time-saving tips in the "Time Saver" boxes throughout this chapter.

As you'll notice, many of the meals in this plan call for fat-free, low-fat, or high-protein foods. What exactly does that mean? To give you a clear picture, here is what to look for when shopping for these products:

- **High-protein cereals:** At least 8 grams of protein and 3 grams of fiber per serving. The Overnight Diet's top picks are Kashi Go Lean (13 grams of protein, 10 grams of fiber), Nature's Path Optimum line of cereals (10 grams of protein, 5 grams of fiber), and Special K Protein (10 grams of protein, 3 grams of fiber).
- **Sugar-free:** Less than 0.5 grams of sugar per serving. Contains no ingredient that is sugar. Look for "No Added Sugars" and "Without Added Sugars" labels.
- **Low-sugar yogurt:** 12 grams of sugar or less.
- **Fat-free:** Less than 0.5 grams of fat per serving. Contains no ingredient that is a fat.
- **Low-fat (1%):** 3 grams of fat or less.
- **Low-sodium:** Less than 140 milligrams of sodium per serving.
- **No-Sodium:** Less than 5 milligrams of sodium per serving.

Benefit from your bottomless buffet. The bottomless buffet of fruits and nonstarchy veggies can replace any of the snack suggestions and is always something you can turn to when you feel hungry. Always keep your favorite fruits and veggies on hand for these times. Trim, wash, and store all fresh veggies for the week at the same time on your R&R day. Store lettuce in a breathable bag in the crisper and all others in a large bowl of water in the fridge. This keeps them just-picked fresh until you're ready to eat them. Also make individual snack bags of veggies so you can just grab and go in the morning.

Week 1, Day 1

1-Day Power Up

Welcome to your first 1-Day Power Up. You may be feeling a bit unsure about what to expect, but just take a look at these enticing, mouthwatering, jumbo smoothies. Each recipe will fill you up and prime your body to burn more fat all day—and all night—long. So cast aside any sense of hesitation and dive right in to rev up rapid weight loss. (Find more recipes at OvernightDiet.org.)

Breakfast: Banana Latte Smoothie, page 139
Kickstart your day with a smoothie so delicious it belongs on the menu of your favorite coffeehouse.

Lunch: Orange Zest Smoothie, page 144
This zesty citrus explosion is like sunshine in a blender—who knew a smoothie lunch could taste so sinfully delicious?

Dinner: Green Apple Goddess Smoothie, page 141
Jazzy pops of tangy green apple dotted with hints of sweetness fill you up completely. No hunger here as you complete your first 1-Day Power Up.

Time Saver

Consider making tomorrow's Spicy Chicken and White Bean Chili and the following day's Hot Black-Eyed Pea Soup today. Chili and soup usually taste better after the flavors have had a chance to blend. Make extra and freeze in preportioned storage containers for quick and easy meals at a later date.

Here's the Skinny

Be generous with the veggies in your smoothies. You won't even taste them, and their high-fiber content bulks up the volume so you will get full faster and stay that way longer.

Week 1, Day 2

6-Day Fuel Up

Breakfast: Crust-less Quiche, page 149
  Grapefruit sections
  ½ whole-wheat bagel thin (I like Lender's)
  1 cup fat-free Greek-style yogurt
  Coffee or tea with fat-free milk and Truvia or Splenda
Snack: Baby carrots with Toasted Cumin Yogurt Dip, page 208
Lunch: Spicy Chicken and White Bean Chili, page 177
  Salad with baby spinach, Mandarin orange slices,
  1 tablespoon slivered almonds, fat-free dressing
  ½ cup cooked brown rice
Snack: Grapes
Dinner: Crusty Oven-Fried Fish, page 186
  Roasted Garlic Cauliflower Mash, page 198
  1 cup green beans
Dessert: ½ cup frozen fat-free yogurt (I like Edy's Slow
  Churned)
  3 fat-free ginger snaps (I like Newman's Own Organics)
Snack: Blueberries and pineapple chunks

Week 1, Day 3

6-Day Fuel Up

Breakfast: 1 cup high-protein, high-fiber cereal (I like Kashi
  Go-Lean)
  Sliced bananas

1 cup fat-free milk

Coffee or tea with fat-free milk and Truvia or Splenda

Snack: Kiwi fruit and strawberry slices

Lunch: Hot Black-Eyed Pea Soup, page 165

Steamed broccoli with lemon

Snack: Apple wedges with fat-free dip

Dinner: 8 ounces ham steak, sautéed in a nonstick pan with olive oil spray

Swiss chard with garlic and parsley, sautéed

Rice Pilaf, page 198

Dessert: 1 cup fat-free yogurt

1 chocolate chip cookie, 2-inch diameter

Snack: Frozen peaches, thawed

Here's the Skinny

How do you eat just one chocolate chip cookie? If you buy an entire box of cookies and nibble on just one of them, then you have to try to ignore the tempting siren call of the rest of those tasty treats in the cupboard, and you know how impossible that is. Having junk food or treats in the house is one of the most common reasons why people fall off a healthy eating plan. It's best to keep trigger foods out of your kitchen. If you want a cookie, buy *one* small cookie from your grocery store bakery. Don't buy a whole box—even though they're cheaper that way—and try to convince yourself that you will have the willpower to eat just one of them. You won't.

Enlist the help of your friends and family for situations like these. Here are a few tricks:

- Split the cost of a box with a friend, take one cookie, and give the rest of the box to your pal. Ask her to dole them out to you according to a preapproved schedule.
- Buy a box, take one cookie, and ask your spouse to take the rest of them to his or her place of work.
- If you prefer homemade cookies, make a small amount of dough, divide it into individual cookie portions, and store

them in the freezer. When it's your "cookie night," take out
one, bake it, and savor the fresh-baked flavor.

- Go for a 100-calorie snack pack that comes with tiny cookies.
  You'll get the satisfaction of eating more than one cookie,
  but because they are so small, they won't do a lot of damage.

Time Saver

Soak black beans today for tomorrow's Black Bean, Corn, and Quinoa
Salad. Rinse and drain soaked beans and add fresh water for cooking
to reduce gas. Tease out some "me time" later in the week by cooking extra beans today for breakfast on Week 1, Day 5, and dinner
on Week 1, Day 7. Refrigerate until needed. Or simply can it! When
you're short on time, opt for low-sodium canned beans rather than
dried beans. You'll get all the flavor and all the health benefits without all that prep time needed to soak and cook dried beans.

Week 1, Day 4

6-Day Fuel Up

Breakfast: Egg and Spinach Omelet, page 151
  ½ grapefruit, lightly toasted under the broiler
  1 slice whole-grain toast
  Coffee or tea with fat-free milk and Truvia or Splenda
Snack: Sliced pears with fat-free dip
Lunch: Black Bean, Corn, and Quinoa Salad, page 193
  4 ounces sautéed chicken strips
  Carrot slices, cooked
Snack: Frozen mango, thawed
Dinner: 8 ounces pan-seared wild salmon (liberally sprinkle
  with freshly ground pepper before cooking)
  Avocado, Fennel, and Citrus Salad, page 191
  ½ cup spinach, sautéed with cooking spray

Dessert: Brownie sundae with:
Chocolate brownie, 2-inch square
½ cup frozen fat-free yogurt
1 tablespoon fat-free whipped cream
Snack: 1 small handful of mixed dried cranberries and raisins

---

Here's the Skinny

Dried fruit is created by removing most of the water content from the fresh fruit. Dried fruit retains most of its nutritional content and dietary fiber. But the packaged varieties sold on store shelves are often infused with some form of sugar to add sweetness, and they are more energy dense than their fresh fruit counterparts. For example, 1 cup of fresh grapes has 104 calories, but 1 cup of raisins packs 434 calories. Because of this, you should limit dried fruits to no more than one small handful a day.

Time Saver

Get a jump on tomorrow—cook an extra 4-ounce salmon fillet tonight for tomorrow's lunch. For complete doneness, cook salmon 4 minutes on each side.

Week 1, Day 5

6-Day Fuel Up

Breakfast: Black Bean Quesadilla, page 148
1 medium orange
Coffee or tea with fat-free milk and Truvia or Splenda
Snack: Baked Cinnamon Apples, page 192
Lunch: 4 ounces pan-seared wild salmon
Oven-roasted cauliflower with olive oil and black pepper
½ cup Spicy Peanut Noodles, page 163

Snack: Pineapple slices
Dinner: Fiery Barbecue Pulled Pork, page 181
  Frozen green beans, cooked
  Broccoli, steamed
Dessert: Lemon Cheesecake Parfait, page 214
Snack: Grapes

Here's the Skinny

Don't wait until you're feeling hungry to prepare your snacks lest you feel tempted to eat off your meal plan. Bake your apples and prep your pineapple while getting ready for your day, if you didn't already do it on your R&R day. Having your snacks ready and waiting helps keep you on track so the weight will keep coming off.

Week 1, Day 6

6-Day Fuel Up

Breakfast: 1 slice low-fat turkey bacon (I like Oscar Mayer Louis Rich)
  1 egg, poached
  Medium orange
  1 whole-wheat bagel thin (I like Lender's)
  1 cup fat-free yogurt
  Coffee or tea with fat-free milk and Truvia or Splenda
Snack: Star fruit
Lunch: Beefy Mushroom Burgers, page 179
  Side salad with fat-free dressing
  1 cup fat-free milk
Snack: Cherries
Dinner: Zesty Broccoli Slaw Salad with Chicken, page 179
Dessert: Apple Cranberry Crisp, page 210
Snack: Carrot and celery sticks

Week 1, Day 7

6-Day Fuel Up

Breakfast: 2 poached eggs
    Sliced banana
    1 whole-grain frozen waffle
    1 cup fat-free yogurt (atop waffle)
    Coffee or tea with fat-free milk and Truvia or Splenda
Snack: Frozen mixed fruit cups
Lunch: Italian "Sausage" Pizza, page 160
    Mesclun lettuce mix, tomatoes, cucumbers, purple onion
    slices, 1 tablespoon fat-free Italian salad dressing
Snack: Blueberries
Dinner: Black Bean and Chicken Chili, page 170
    Spinach and garlic, sautéed
Dessert: Peachy Oat Crumble, page 216
Snack: Unsweetened applesauce (I like Langers)

Time Saver

Say hello to a quick and easy day! Use the reserved black beans from Week 1, Day 4, and use Boboli 100% whole-wheat pizza crust for a fast and easy pizza lunch.

Week 2, Day 1

1-Day Power Up

Congratulations—you've already completed your first week! By now, the number on your scale is going down, and you're motivated to keep it heading in that direction. Your second smoothie day will stoke your body's fat-burning engines while you get to enjoy a little R&R.

Breakfast: Crispy Apple Smoothie, page 140
    Awaken to a honey crisp apple smoothie teeming with juicy
    bursts of citrus! Protein powder, fruits, and veggies guarantee
    boundless energy and enthusiasm to get your day off to a
    great start.
Lunch: Mexican Chocolate Banana Swirl Smoothie, page 143
    Scents of cinnamon and chocolate commingle in your glass to
    delight the senses and provide total satisfaction.
Dinner: Green Machine Smoothie, page 142
    End your day with a savory smoothie that's voluminous in
    flavor and fullness.

Time Saver

Make Overnight Power Oatmeal, page 155, today for tomorrow's
breakfast. In the morning, just add the protein powder to the precooked porridge.

Week 2, Day 2

6-Day Fuel Up

Breakfast: Overnight Power Oatmeal, page 155
    Coffee or tea with fat-free milk and Truvia or Splenda
Snack: Stewed Golden Delicious apples with cinnamon
Lunch: Tuna wrap sandwich with:
    Mediterranean Tuna Salad, page 188
    Whole-wheat lavash (I like Joseph's Flax, Oat Bran, & Whole
    Wheat Square Lavash)
    Lettuce, tomatoes, sprouts, purple or sweet yellow onion
Snack: Plums
Dinner: 8 ounces roast London broil
    Black Bean, Corn, and Quinoa Salad, page 193

Salad of green lettuces, shredded carrots, radishes, and fat-free dressing
Dessert: Apple Cinnamon Brown Rice Pudding, page 209
Snack: Clementines

Here's the Skinny

Choose the sprouts you like best. In case you aren't familiar with them, sprouts are germinated seeds that are rich in vitamins and minerals, amino acids, protein, and dietary fiber. Alfalfa sprouts are the most widely recognized type, but there are many other varieties, all with varying amounts of protein and nutritional values. Here are some of the nutritional benefits of the most common types of sprouts.

- Alfalfa sprouts: 35 percent protein, more chlorophyll than spinach or kale, as much carotene as carrots.
- Mung bean sprouts: 20 percent protein, great source of vitamin C, B vitamins, and vitamin K.
- Lentil sprouts: 25 percent protein, high in folate, great source of vitamin C and B vitamins.

Week 2, Day 3

6-Day Fuel Up

Breakfast: Smoked Salmon and Egg Open-Faced Sandwich, page 157
Cucumbers and yogurt dip
Apple wedges
Coffee or tea with fat-free milk and Truvia or Splenda
Snack: 1 handful Craisins
Lunch: Cashew Chicken Salad with Cilantro Dressing, page 171
6 whole-grain crackers (I like Wasa Crisp Bread Crackers)
Snack: Cantaloupe cubes

Dinner: 8 ounces baked chicken breast
　　Carrot Soup with North African Spices, page 164
　　Fennel, Apple, and Arugula Salad, page 194
Dessert: Sugar-free Jell-O
　　1 tablespoon fat-free whipped topping
Snack: Strawberries sprinkled with sugar substitute

Week 2, Day 4

6-Day Fuel Up

Breakfast: Breakfast Taco, page 148
　　Persimmon
　　Coffee or tea with fat-free milk and Truvia or Splenda
Snack: Pan-seared banana slices
Lunch: Hot Black-Eyed Pea Soup, page 165
　　Side salad of tomato cubes, cucumber chunks, and purple
　　onion slices with fat-free Italian dressing
　　½ cup asparagus spears
Snack: Apple slices
Dinner: Spaghetti and Meat Sauce, page 162
　　1 cup cooked spinach
Dessert: Mug of sugar-free hot cocoa (I like CocoaVia)
　　1 tablespoon fat-free whipped topping
　　Sprinkle of cinnamon
Snack: 1 ounce low-fat cheddar cheese
　　6 whole-wheat crackers

Week 2, Day 5

6-Day Fuel Up

Breakfast: 1 cup cooked quinoa
　　½ avocado, sliced

1 sausage patty (I like Morningstar Farms)
½ cup fat-free cottage cheese
Coffee or tea with fat-free milk and Truvia or Splenda
Snack: Sliced bananas
Lunch: Magician Salad with Ahi Tuna, page 187
Snack: Grapefruit, sectioned
Dinner: 8 ounces baked chicken breast
Roasted Garlic Cauliflower Mash, page 198
Dessert: 1 cup fat-free yogurt
2 Granola Plum Mini-Muffin Pastries page 212
Snack: Baby carrots with Toasted Cumin Yogurt Dip, page 208

Here's the Skinny

Enjoying an evening dessert that is filled with fiber, such as Granola Plum Mini-Muffin Pastries, ensures your GI tract will be running smoothly the next day.

Time Saver

Let your salad dressing do double duty as a dipping sauce for veggies. Make extra Sesame Miso Dressing to use throughout the week for your bottomless buffet of veggies.

Week 2, Day 6

6-Day Fuel Up

Breakfast: Egg and Veggie Scramble, page 152
Mandarin orange slices and ½ cup dry old-fashioned oatmeal mixed into 1 cup fat-free Greek yogurt
Coffee or tea with fat-free milk and Truvia or Splenda
Snack: Vanilla Poached Pears, page 199

Lunch: Healthy Layered Vegetable Salad with Bacon, page 174
4 ounces grilled chicken breast
Snack: Raspberry and blackberry mix
Dinner: 8 ounces filet mignon
Sautéed zucchini and yellow summer squash
½ cup farro, cooked
Dessert: ½ cup fat-free ice cream (I like Edy's Slow Churned)
1 Figgy Cookie, page 211
Snack: Grapes

Time Saver

Farro takes about 50 minutes to cook. Make double or triple the amount you need, then divide into individual serving sizes and freeze in freezer bowls.

Week 2, Day 7

6-Day Fuel Up

Breakfast: Garden Veggie Frittata, page 153
1 slice whole-wheat toast
1 cup fat-free Greek yogurt
Coffee or tea with fat-free milk and Truvia or Splenda
Snack: Tangerines
Lunch: Chicken Pasta with Fresh Summer Vegetables, page 160
Carrots and celery, raw and sliced
Snack: Mango slices
Dinner: Old-Fashioned Beef Stew, page 183
Salad with baby spinach, Mandarin orange slices, fat-free dressing
Dessert: 1 cup Grandma's Low-Fat Chocolate Pudding, page 212
1 tablespoon fat-free whipped topping
1 teaspoon candied ginger pieces
Snack: Tangerines

Week 3, Day 1

1-Day Power Up

After two full weeks, you are beginning to see just how fast you can burn fat and lose weight with this combo diet. By now, you may be noticing that your jeans don't fit as snugly as they used to, you have more energy, and you don't feel as hungry as you used to. And you're undoubtedly looking forward to today's 1-Day Power Up so you can lose up to 2 more pounds overnight. Rest assured, you'll be doing it in delicious style.

Breakfast: Enchanted Blueberry Smoothie, page 141
   Rich, thick, and brimming with vibrant flavor, this smoothie is packed with the powerful antioxidant power of blueberries.
Lunch: Delightfully Spicy Smoothie, page 140
   Spice up your day with a tangy smoothie that is sure to tantalize your taste buds and keep you cruising through the afternoon.
Dinner: Piña Colada Island Smoothie, page 145
   Celebrate today's ending with a piña colada–style smoothie that puts you in the vacation mood, thanks to sweet pineapple and creamy coconut.

Week 3, Day 2

6-Day Fuel Up

Breakfast: Mexican Pita with Shrimp, page 154
   Grapes
   Coffee or tea with fat-free milk and Truvia or Splenda
Snack: Apple slices
Lunch: Spicy Tuna Delight, page 190
   1 cup carrots, steamed with 1 teaspoon non-trans-fat buttery spread (I like Earth Balance)
Snack: Sliced bananas

Dinner: Braised Tenderloin Cutlets in Mushroom and Red Wine Sauce, page 180
  Side salad with 1 tablespoon Lemon Caper Vinaigrette, page 204
  ½ cup quinoa, cooked
Dessert: "On the Beam" Brownie, page 216
Snack: Cherries

Week 3, Day 3

6-Day Fuel Up

Breakfast: Sausage and Egg Scramble, page 156
  ½ cup fat-free cottage cheese
  Coffee or tea with fat-free milk and Truvia or Splenda
Snack: Plums
Lunch: 1 turkey wrap with:
  4 ounces turkey
  1 slice low-fat cheese
  Whole-wheat lavash (I like Joseph's Flax, Oat Bran & Whole Wheat Square Lavash)
  Lettuce, tomato, onion, pickles, sprouts, mustard
  Sautéed French-style green beans
Snack: Canned fruit (in its own juice)
Dinner: Rosemary Pork Roast, page 184
  Mesclun mix salad with Honey Garlic Balsamic Vinaigrette, page 204
Dessert: Lemon Custard with Fresh Blueberry Sauce, page 215
Snack: Melon balls

Time Saver
Cook an extra 8 ounces of the Rosemary Pork Roast to save for Week 3, Day 5.

Week 3, Day 4

6-Day Fuel Up

Breakfast: Spicy Tofu Scramble, page 158
   Coffee or tea with fat-free milk and Truvia or Splenda
Snack: Strawberry slices sprinkled with sugar substitute
   (optional)
Lunch: Tuna salad sandwich with:
   Tuna salad (3 ounces water-packed tuna, 1 hard-boiled egg,
   2 tablespoons fat-free mayonnaise, salt and pepper to taste)
   Sliced tomato, lettuce, sprouts, purple onion
   1 slice whole-grain bread
Snack: Baked banana slices with just a drizzle of maple syrup
Dinner: Shepherd's Pie with Chicken, page 176
Dessert: ½ cup fat-free ice cream (I like Edy's Slow Churned)
   2 fat-free ginger snaps (I like Newman's Own Organics)
   1 tablespoon fat-free whipped topping
Snack: Apples with Creamy Peanut Dip, page 190

Here's the Skinny

Don't miss out on the health benefits and high-protein content of yogurt just because you have trouble digesting dairy products. If you experience gas, bloating, or stomach pains after eating these foods, it may be due to an inability to process lactose, a type of sugar found in milk and dairy products. This is called lactose intolerance. But there's hope. Certain dairy products are naturally lower in lactose, including hard, aged cheeses, such as cheddar, Swiss, and parmesan; cottage cheese; and yogurts with live and active cultures. In addition, most supermarkets carry lactose-reduced or lactose-free dairy products, which minimize any digestive problems. You can also try probiotics to ease symptoms of lactose intolerance. Kefir is a natural probiotic drink, similar to liquid yogurt, that keeps your GI system running smoothly. You can also take a supplement, such as Lactaid, that provides the enzyme, lactase, needed by your body to digest dairy.

Time Saver

Make Celery Root Rémoulade tonight for tomorrow's lunch to allow the flavor to enhance.

Week 3, Day 5

6-Day Fuel Up

Breakfast: Diana's Magnificent Hearty Pancakes, page 150
  1 cup fat-free yogurt (spread on pancake)
  1 apple and 1 pear stewed with cinnamon, cloves, and
  nutmeg (atop yogurt layer)
  Coffee or tea with fat-free milk and Truvia or Splenda
Snack: Bananas, strawberries, and blueberries
Lunch: 4 ounces oven-baked chicken breast
  Celery Root Rémoulade, page 194
  1 whole-grain roll
Snack: Orange segments
Dinner: Rosemary Pork Roast, page 184
  Zucchini and yellow squash medley, steamed
Dessert: Grapes and Walnuts with Lemon Sour Cream Sauce,
  page 213
Snack: Carrot coins, cucumber slices, and celery sticks

Time Saver

Using the Rosemary Pork Roast you cooked on Week 3, Day 3, means dinner will be ready in a flash.

Week 3, Day 6

6-Day Fuel Up

Breakfast: Sausage and Egg Scramble, page 156
  1 cup low-fat kefir
  Coffee or tea with fat-free milk and Truvia or Splenda

Snack: Stewed apples with cinnamon and a sprinkle of sugar
substitute
Lunch: Lemon Roasted Salmon, page 187
Asparagus spears, grilled
Quick and Easy Lemon Pasta, page 161
Snack: Melon cubes
Dinner: Thai Chicken Noodle Soup, page 167
Thai Chicken Salad, page 178
Dessert: Grilled Fruit with Balsamic Syrup, page 214
Snack: 1 handful dried fruit mixture

Here's the Skinny

Why lemon salmon *and* lemon pasta today? When you eat meals containing similar flavors, it allows for something called taste saturation, which makes you feel full faster.

Week 3, Day 7

6-Day Fuel Up

Breakfast: 2 poached eggs
1 cup fat-free yogurt
Coffee or tea with fat-free milk and Truvia or Splenda
Snack: Pomegranate (peel the pomegranate, then eat it kernel
by kernel for a long-lasting snack)
Lunch: 4 ounces grilled shrimp
Green beans, sautéed
½ cup whole-wheat couscous
Snack: Raw cauliflower with Savory Yogurt Dip, page 206
Dinner: Indian Spiced Chicken, page 175
Rice Pilaf, page 198
Spinach side salad with fat-free salad dressing
Dessert: ½ cup fat-free frozen strawberry yogurt (I like Edy's
Slow Churned)

1 slice angel food cake
Sliced strawberries
Snack: Apple slices

Week 4, Day 1

1-Day Power Up

After just 21 days, you should be looking leaner, feeling stronger, and bursting with more energy than ever before. Give yourself a pat on the back! Then spark overnight weight loss again with a trio of smoothies that will make you feel like you're on vacation. You deserve it.

Breakfast: Morning Sunshine Smoothie, page 144
The sweetness of mango and banana in this zingy treat immediately puts you in vacation mode. Is there a better way to start your day?
Lunch: Tropical Medley Smoothie, page 147
This delightful drink is bursting with flavors from the islands—mango, coconut, and banana—that will transport you to a tropical paradise. Sip away on this supersized smoothie all afternoon.
Dinner: Kale Margarita Smoothie, page 142
What a perfect way to wind down a vacation day. Enjoy a different kind of margarita that's smooth and sweet and is guaranteed to leave you feeling lively and energetic tomorrow morning.

Week 4, Day 2

6-Day Fuel Up

Breakfast: Spicy Egg Scramble, page 157
1 cup fat-free yogurt
Coffee or tea with fat-free milk and Truvia or Splenda

Snack: Red bell peppers and French-style green beans with fat-free dressing as dip

Lunch: Extra-Healthy Spinach Salad with Turkey, page 173

Snack: Frozen mango, strawberries, and banana bits sweetened with a touch of agave nectar

Dinner: Chicken and Veggie Stir-Fry, page 172
½ cup brown basmati rice

Dessert: 1 cup low-fat tapioca pudding (I like Whole Foods or Healthy Choice)
1 biscotti

Snack: Tangerines

Week 4, Day 3

6-Day Fuel Up

Breakfast: Egg and Spinach Omelet, page 151
Orange, sliced
½ whole-wheat sesame bagel, toasted
Toasted Cumin Yogurt Dip, page 208
Coffee or tea with fat-free milk and Truvia or Splenda

Snack: Strawberries, blueberries, raspberries, and blackberries drizzled with balsamic vinegar and a pinch of brown sugar (optional)

Lunch: Vegetable Stir-Fry, page 184 with 4 ounces pork

Snack: Cucumber slices, tomato wedges, purple onion rings with Savory Yogurt Dip, page 206

Dinner: 8 ounces filet mignon
Spinach, sautéed with garlic
Mushrooms, sautéed
½ cup farro cooked

Dessert: Cherries with Ricotta and Toasted Almonds, page 210

Snack: Mandarin oranges, drain first if canned

Time Saver

Prepare Baked Burritos and Parmesan Tomatoes tonight for tomorrow's dinner. Cover with foil and place in the fridge. When you're ready to bake, let them sit at room temperature for 30 minutes before popping in the oven.

Week 4, Day 4

6-Day Fuel Up

Breakfast: 1 cup high-protein, high-fiber cereal (I like Kashi GoLean)
1 egg, soft-boiled
1 cup fat-free milk
Applesauce, unsweetened (I like Langers or Mott's)
Coffee or tea with fat-free milk and Truvia or Splenda
Snack: Mango and pineapple slushy (blend frozen fruit with ice and eat with a spoon)
Lunch: Apple Tuna Roll-Up, page 185
Snack: Fresh figs
Dinner: Baked Chicken Burritos, page 169
Baked Parmesan Tomato, page 192
Dessert: 1 cup low-fat chocolate pudding (I like Whole Foods or Jell-O)
3 fat-free ginger snaps (I like Newman's Own Organics)
Snack: Grapefruit sections

Week 4, Day 5

6-Day Fuel Up

Breakfast: Oat Pudding with Chocolate and Lime, page 154
2 scrambled eggs
Coffee or tea with fat-free milk and Truvia or Splenda

Snack: Baby carrots
Lunch: Mac and Cheese Cauliflower, page 197
    4 ounces grilled chicken breast
    Swiss chard, sautéed
Snack: Apple slices
Dinner: Pan-Fried Wild Salmon and Mustard Sauce, page 189
    Japanese Spinach Salad, page 196
    Miso soup
Dessert: 1 cup fat-free steamed milk with nutmeg
    Graham cracker, 1 full sheet (I like Nabisco Honey Maid
    Original Grahams)
Snack: Peaches

Week 4, Day 6

6-Day Fuel Up

Breakfast: 2-egg veggie omelet (with liberal doses of spinach,
    mushrooms, tomatoes, and onions)
    1 slice whole-grain toast
    2 tablespoons natural peanut butter
    Coffee or tea with fat-free milk and Truvia or Splenda
Snack: Cherries
    1 cup fat-free chocolate milk
Lunch: White Chicken Pizza, page 163
    Large Caesar salad with fat-free dressing and no croutons
Snack: Grapes
Dinner: 8 ounces grilled steak
    1 cup roasted cauliflower
    1 cup roasted asparagus spears
Dessert: Sundae with:
    ½ cup fat-free frozen yogurt
    1 tablespoon fat-free chocolate syrup (I like Hershey's)
    1 tablespoon fat-free whipped topping
Snack: Fresh veggie sticks and Toasted Cumin Yogurt Dip,
    page 208

Week 4, Day 7

6-Day Fuel Up

Breakfast: Egg and Veggie Scramble, page 152
½ cup dry oatmeal, cooked
1 tablespoon raisins
1 cup sugar-free hot cocoa (I like CocoaVia)
Coffee or tea with fat-free milk and Truvia or Splenda
Snack: Sliced bananas with a sprinkle of cinnamon, toast lightly
Lunch: Tomato basil soup, canned
Meatloaf, page 182, sandwich with:
2 slices light whole-grain bread
Condiments: mustard, horseradish, sliced sweet onions,
pickles, lettuce, tomatoes, capers
Snack: Cucumbers, tomatoes, and purple onions with fat-free
Italian dressing for dipping
Dinner: Berry, Jicama, and Apple Salad, page 193
8 ounces roast turkey breast
Dessert: Brownie sundae with:
1 chocolate brownie, 2-inch square
½ cup frozen fat-free yogurt
1 tablespoon fat-free whipped cream
Snack: Strawberries

CHAPTER 7

1-Day Power Up Recipes

The smoothie recipes here and in Appendix C will keep you feeling refreshed, energized, and satisfied as you burn fat and boost your overall health. Diana Cullum-Dugan, lead nutritionist at the Nutrition and Weight Management Center at Boston Medical Center, took on the challenge to help come up with the smoothie recipes to include in this book, and it was a tall order. To maximize the 1-Day Power Up's potential to jump-start weight loss, each smoothie had to meet some very exacting specifications, which included:

- Providing protein to maintain lean muscle
- Containing plenty of fiber to promote smooth digestion and to keep you feeling pleasantly satiated for hours
- Using wholesome, good-for-your-health foods
- Using everyday ingredients you can easily find
- Taking less than 3 minutes to make
- And most important, being undeniably, unequivocally, lip-smackingly delicious

The smoothies you'll find here succeeded on every count beyond all expectations. Of course, they all underwent rigorous taste testing. Smoothie taste-testing day turned out to be a real favorite at the Center. Week after week, doctors, nurses, and support staff members would all crowd around to get a taste of the samples. The funny thing is that everybody had very different preferences, but the

136

smoothies offered something amazing for each one. Some people fell in love with the refreshing fruity varieties such as Enchanted Blueberry and Crispy Apple. One of the nurses always went back for seconds of the savory flavors, such as Delightfully Spicy, which has a little kick to it. And one of the assistants couldn't stop raving about the thick, creamy dessert-like smoothies with hints of chocolate (Spa Crazy Chocolate) or peanut butter (Peanut Butter Cup).

You'll find something you love, too. Whether you gravitate toward spicy, savory, or sweet, you'll discover sinlessly delicious recipes to suit your taste. Some patients like a fruity creation in the morning, something a little more savory for lunch, and a sweet treat in the evening. You are encouraged to aim for variety by choosing three separate smoothies throughout the day rather than sticking with the same one morning, noon, and night.

Dapper Apple

Protein: 1 serving protein powder (Physicians Protein Smoothies Base Mix, or whey, or soy)

2 medium apples, cored, peeled, and chopped

2 cups spinach

1 cup unsweetened almond milk

1 cup ice cubes

Banana Blast-Off

Protein: 1 serving protein powder (Physicians Protein Smoothies Base Mix, or whey, or soy)

2 medium bananas

2 cups kale

½–1 cup water

1 cup ice cubes

Figure-Friendly Fennel

Protein: 1 serving protein powder (Physicians Protein Smoothies Base Mix, or whey, or soy)

2 cups fennel bulb
2 large oranges, peeled and sectioned
½ cup nonfat milk
½–1 cup water
1 cup ice cubes

Mighty Fine Mango

Protein: 1 serving protein powder (Physicians Protein Smoothies Base
    Mix, or whey, or soy)
2 cups mango
2 cups spinach
1 cup coconut water
1 cup ice cubes

All of these smoothies are big in size, flavor, and fat-burning power. What makes them even better is that you can whip them up in mere moments. Grab a handful of ingredients, toss them in a blender, and press a button. What could be easier? If you're a busy parent or constantly on the go, you need something that's lightning fast to prepare. You won't find anything that's quicker or easier to make that will give you the overnight results you want. They're economical, too, so they won't lighten your wallet much while lightening your weight. The recipes that follow list ingredients; these simple instructions apply to every one of them.

To see how simple it is to make these tasty creations, check out OvernightDiet.org for video demonstrations. If you want even more, visit the website or Dr. Caroline Apovian's Facebook page, where you'll find additional recipes from patients and from other readers. Feel free to join the conversation and share your own recipes there, too.

Important note: You do *not* have to adjust the protein amounts in the smoothie recipes to your DPR. The DPR is strictly for the 6-Day Fuel Up.

Another important note: In recipes that call for milk, both here and in Chapter 8, you should stick to fat-free or 1% if you're using cow's milk. Always feel free to substitute with unsweetened almond milk or soy milk if you prefer.

Banana Latte

Everybody loves a latte. This banana-flavored coffee smoothie is so good, and you definitely can't get it at your local coffee shop. Enjoy it as a healthy pick-me-up any time of day.

Protein: 1 serving protein powder (Physicians Protein Smoothies Base Mix, or whey, or soy)

1 cup fat-free milk

¾ cup strong black coffee (decaf is okay)

1 banana, sliced

1 cup ice cubes

Blueberry Freeze

Frozen blueberries and fresh banana add creamy thickness to this fruity delight.

Protein: 1 cup fat-free plain Greek yogurt

1 banana, sliced

½–1 cup water

1½ teaspoons ground flaxseeds

1 cup frozen blueberries

Help! My Smoothie's Too Thick

If your smoothie comes out thicker than you would like, simply add a little water to give it a thinner consistency. In general, if you prefer a smoothie that's closer to a juice in consistency, use fresh produce rather than frozen, and use water rather than ice.

Help! My Smoothie's Too Watery

If you've made your smoothie and it comes out thinner than you would like, just add small amounts of ice until it reaches the thickness you desire. If you tend to prefer a thicker smoothie, try using frozen fruits and veggies. That really helps create a thick and creamy consistency.

Remember, for any of these recipes, you can use fresh *or* frozen fruits and veggies.

California Dreaming

If you're dreaming about being ready for bikini season, this peachy smoothie will help you make that dream a reality.

Protein: 1 cup fat-free plain Greek yogurt

1 cup sliced peaches

1 cup strawberries

1 tablespoon ground flaxseeds

3 cups ice cubes

Cherry Jubilee

Delectable cherries of your choosing, such as deep-red Bing or yellowy-red Rainier, make this a celebration-worthy smoothie.

Protein: 1 serving protein powder (Physicians Protein Smoothies Base Mix, or whey, or soy)

1 banana, sliced

1 cup pitted cherries

2 cups water

1 handful spinach

Crispy Apple

Give this juicy smoothie a twist by going for a tart Granny Smith apple, or make a sweeter version with Red Gold, Red Delicious, Honeycrisp, or Fuji apples.

Protein: 1 serving protein powder (Physicians Protein Smoothies Base Mix, or whey, or soy)

1 cup water

1 apple, cored, seeded, and quartered

1 medium orange, peeled and quartered

2 handfuls spinach

1 medium carrot, peeled and sliced

Delightfully Spicy

Filled with spicy notes (arugula peppers the palate), this tangy smoothie is sure to spice up your day. Add crushed red pepper flakes for a more intense bite.

Protein: 1 serving protein powder (Physicians Protein Smoothies Base Mix, or whey, or soy)

1 large bell pepper (red, orange, or yellow)

1 orange, peeled and quartered

1 celery stalk

1 cup arugula

1½ cups water

¼ teaspoon crushed red pepper flakes (optional)

Enchanted Blueberry

You'll be enchanted by this blueberry-infused treat that sneaks in some good-for-you veggies.

Protein: 1 serving protein powder (Physicians Protein Smoothies Base Mix, or whey, or soy)

¾ cup fat-free blueberry yogurt

2 handfuls spinach

1 cup blueberries

2 cups ice cubes

Figtastic

Fantastic fiber-rich figs provide the foundation for this one-of-a-kind creation, while hints of cinnamon and vanilla give it even more flair.

Protein: 1 serving protein powder (Physicians Protein Smoothies Base Mix, or whey, or soy)

4–5 figs (preferably fresh, but dried are okay, too)

½ cup red seedless grapes

1 cup water

1 cup ice cubes

½ teaspoon ground cinnamon

½ teaspoon vanilla

Green Apple Goddess

This smoothie is almost like having a whole fruit basket in a blender.

Protein: 1 serving protein powder (Physicians Protein Smoothies Base Mix, or whey, or soy)

1 Granny Smith apple, cored, seeded, and quartered
½ cup blueberries
½ cup diced pineapple (canned in water or its own juice is okay)
½ cup raspberries
1–2 handfuls spinach
½ head hearts of Romaine lettuce
2 large kale leaves, destemmed and chopped
2 cups water

Green Machine

Going green has never been more delicious! Add in the tomato and the celery stalk, and you just might think you're enjoying a virgin Bloody Mary on the veranda.

Protein: 1 cup fat-free plain Greek yogurt
1 cup ice cubes
1 medium cucumber, peeled and sliced
1 medium carrot, peeled and sliced
1 small tomato, quartered
1 celery stalk, sliced
2 handfuls spinach
Salt and pepper to taste

Kale Margarita

There's nothing like a margarita to make your day. Bitter kale, sweet mango, and succulent coconut water make up for the lack of tequila.

Protein: 1 serving protein powder (Physicians Protein Smoothies Base Mix, or whey, or soy)
1 cup destemmed and chopped kale
1 cup peeled and cubed mango
1½ cups Jordan's Skinny Margarita Mix
½ cup coconut water
1 cup ice

Key Lime Pie

If you love key lime pie (and who doesn't?), you'll love the refreshing goodness of this smoothie. Zesty lime combines with tropical coconut for a taste explosion.

Protein: 1 serving protein powder (Physicians Protein Smoothies Base Mix, or whey, or soy)

2 tablespoons key lime juice (or juice of a regular lime)

2 teaspoons key lime zest (or zest of a regular lime)

½ cup light, unsweetened coconut milk

½ cup water

1 banana, sliced

1 teaspoon agave nectar

1 tablespoon old-fashioned oats, dry

1 teaspoon vanilla

Mango Madness

Bursting with the juicy sweetness of mango, this smoothie also holds a hint of savory in the form of arugula and spinach.

Protein: 1 serving protein powder (Physicians Protein Smoothies Base Mix, or whey, or soy)

1 banana, sliced

1 orange, peeled and quartered

Handful of arugula

2 handfuls spinach

½ cup peaches

1 cup peeled and cubed mango

1–2 cups water

Mexican Chocolate Banana Swirl

Olé! In a Mexican tradition adopted from the Aztec culture, chocolate commingles with cinnamon for a satisfying, spicy creation.

Protein: 1 serving protein powder (Physicians Protein Smoothies Base Mix, or whey, or soy)

1 banana, sliced

1 tablespoon fat-free chocolate syrup (I like Hershey's)

½ teaspoon cinnamon
1 cup fat-free milk
1 cup ice

Mint Melody

Refreshingly cool and highly flavorful, this minty smoothie perks you up and puts a little pep in your step.

Protein: 1 serving protein powder (Physicians Protein Smoothies Base Mix, or whey, or soy)
1 cup pineapple, cubed (canned in water or its own juice is okay)
1 banana, sliced
1 cup mint leaves
1 cup water

Morning Sunshine

Nothing says "good morning" like sunshine. Sweetness pulsates from dried plums, mango, and banana. You can have your morning sunshine any time of day—for breakfast, lunch, or dinner.

Protein: 1 serving protein powder (Physicians Protein Smoothies Base Mix, or whey, or soy)
5 pitted prunes
½ banana, sliced
1 cup peeled and diced mango
2 handfuls spinach

Orange Zest

Juice up your day with America's most popular citrus fruit.

Protein: 1 serving protein powder (Physicians Protein Smoothies Base Mix, or whey, or soy)
Zest of 1 whole orange
1 whole seedless orange, quartered (including the flesh, sections, and pith)
½ banana, sliced
1 Italian plum, pitted (or regular plum)
Juice of 1 whole lemon
3 large Swiss chard leaves, deribbed

Peanut Butter Cup

Ever had a peanut butter cup in a glass? That's what this amazing dessert-like smoothie tastes like.

Protein: 1 cup fat-free plain Greek yogurt

½–1 cup water

1 tablespoon fat-free chocolate syrup

1 tablespoon creamy peanut butter (I like Smuckers All Natural, regular)

1 banana, sliced

Piña Colada Island

When you want something sweet, try this smoothie filled with chunks of pineapple, creamy coconut, and naturally wholesome agave nectar.

Protein: 1 cup fat-free plain Greek yogurt

1 cup pineapple chunks (canned in water or its own juice is okay)

1 banana, sliced

½ teaspoon coconut extract

1 teaspoon agave nectar

1 cup ice to start (add more as needed for consistency)

Punchy Pomegranate

Pomegranates have been heralded for generations for their divine flavor and health benefits.

Protein: 1 serving protein powder (Physicians Protein Smoothies Base Mix, or whey, or soy)

½ cup pomegranate juice

1 handful kale, Swiss chard, or spinach, destemmed if necessary

1 banana, sliced

¼ cup strawberries

1 tablespoon ground flaxseeds

½–1 cup water

Really Green and Clean

Enjoy a delightful blend of sweet freshness and savory goodness that will leave you feeling energized and ready to go.

Protein: 1 serving protein powder (Physicians Protein Smoothies Base
     Mix, or whey, or soy)
1 medium carrot, peeled and sliced
½ medium sweet apple, cored, seeded, and quartered
1 banana, sliced
2 handfuls spinach (or kale, destemmed)
1 cup water to start (add more as needed for consistency)

Spa Crazy Chocolate

You'll go crazy for this chocolate combo—you might think it came from
the local ice cream shop!

Protein: 1 serving protein powder (Physicians Protein Smoothies Base
     Mix, or whey, or soy)
½–1 cup water
½ teaspoon blackstrap molasses (I like Grandma's, which can be found
     in most supermarkets)
2 tablespoons Truvia (or Splenda)
2 tablespoons cocoa powder, unsweetened (I like Now or Hershey's)
1 banana, sliced
1 small carrot, peeled
1 small celery stalk, sliced
1 handful spinach
2 cups ice cubes

Spicy First Date

In the mood for a hint of spice? Savor sweetly delicious, decidedly exotic
dates enveloped in the intoxicating scent of vanilla along with overtones of
ginger, cloves, and chili.

Protein: 1 cup fat-free plain Greek yogurt
4 Medjool (or regular) dates, pitted
1 cup spinach
½–1 cup water
½ teaspoon pure vanilla extract
½–1 teaspoon cinnamon
Pinch each of ground ginger, cloves, nutmeg, chili powder, and ground
     cayenne pepper
1 cup ice

Strawberry Fields

Take just one sip of this smoothie and you'll understand why strawberries are the most popular berry in the world.

Protein: 1 serving protein powder (Physicians Protein Smoothies Base Mix, or whey, or soy)

½ cup strawberries

½ cup water

¼ cup orange juice (pulp or no pulp, freshly squeezed or store-bought)

Tropical Medley

Prepare your taste buds for a mouthwatering mix of island-inspired flavors.

Protein: 1 serving protein powder (Physicians Protein Smoothies Base Mix, or whey, or soy)

1 banana, sliced

½ cup peeled and diced mango

¼ cup light, unsweetened coconut milk

1 cup water

3 handfuls Swiss chard or spinach, deribbed

1 teaspoon vanilla extract

CHAPTER 8

6-Day Fuel Up Recipes

Find more recipes at OvernightDiet.org.

BREAKFASTS

Black Bean Quesadilla

Prep Time: 10 minutes ▪ Cook Time: 5 minutes ▪ Yield: 1 serving ▪ Protein per Serving Toward DPR: 2 ounces

Protein and fiber from legumes and whole grains increase satiety to stave off hunger.

Protein: 2 egg whites, adjust to your DPR
Nonstick cooking spray
1 8-inch whole-wheat tortilla
¼ cup black beans (rinsed and drained well)
2 ounces low-fat Monterey jack cheese, shredded
Salsa, unlimited

Spray a small nonstick skillet with the cooking spray and scramble the egg whites. Spoon the eggs onto the tortilla. Reduce the heat while you top the egg whites with black beans and cheese. Respray the skillet, fold the tortilla in half, and place in the skillet. Over medium-high heat, cook until lightly browned on one side; flip and cook until the cheese has melted. Top with a generous amount of salsa.

Breakfast Taco

Prep Time: 5 minutes ▪ Cook Time: 2 minutes ▪ Yield: 1 serving ▪ Protein per Serving Toward DPR: 2 ounces

Perfect for days when you're short on time, this south of the border breakfast provides a protein boost that keeps you feeling full all morning long.

Protein: 2 eggs, adjust to your DPR

2 8-inch corn tortillas

Salsa, unlimited

1 handful (or more) baby spinach leaves

2 tablespoons shredded 50% or 75% reduced-fat Cheddar cheese

Nonstick cooking spray

Salt and freshly ground pepper to taste

Spread the tortillas with salsa. Layer on baby spinach leaves to your liking, then sprinkle the cheese on top. In a dry skillet, toast the tortillas until the cheese has melted. (If you must, you can heat in the microwave until the cheese is melted, about 30 seconds, or use a toaster oven.) While the tortillas are toasting, spray a small nonstick skillet with cooking spray. Heat the skillet over medium heat, add the eggs, and scramble until cooked through. Divide the scrambled egg between the tortillas. Top with more salsa, if desired, and season to taste with salt and pepper.

> In any recipes that call for eggs, feel free to use egg whites or egg substitute—but don't forget to adjust your ingredient amounts to maintain your DPR. One large egg contains 1 ounce of protein. The equivalent would be the whites of 2 large eggs, or ¼ cup of egg substitute.

Crust-less Quiche

Prep Time: 10–15 minutes ▪ Cook Time: 30 minutes ▪ Yield: 4 servings ▪ Protein per Serving Toward DPR: 2 ounces

Who needs crust? The rich creaminess of eggs and feta cheese mixed with a pop of spinach make this a go-to! Note that if you make this on Monday, you could have three pieces left over to grab and go throughout the week.

Protein: 3 large eggs plus whites of 2 eggs, adjust to your DPR

Protein: 4 ounces sliced ham, diced, adjust to your DPR

Nonstick cooking spray

1 medium onion, finely diced

1 teaspoon olive oil
6 ounces baby spinach
½ cup whole-wheat flour
½ teaspoon baking powder
¼ teaspoon salt
⅛ teaspoon cayenne pepper
1⅓ cups fat-free milk
Salt and freshly ground pepper to taste
½ cup low-fat feta cheese

Preheat the oven to 400°F. Spray a 10-inch pie plate with the cooking spray. In a medium frying pan, cook the diced onion in olive oil until soft, stirring often. Add the spinach and cook until wilted, 1–2 minutes. Set aside.

In a large bowl, whisk together the eggs, egg whites, flour, baking powder, salt, and cayenne pepper. Then, whisk in the milk just until blended. Stir in the spinach-onion mixture and the ham. Season with salt and pepper to taste.

Pour the mixture into the pie plate, top with feta cheese, and bake for 25 minutes or until the center is set and the edge is golden brown.

Let set for 5 minutes before slicing and serving.

Diana's Magnificent Hearty Pancakes

Prep Time: 10 minutes ▪ Cook Time: 20 minutes ▪ Yield: 12 5-inch pancakes, serving size: 2 pancakes ▪ Protein per Serving Toward DPR: 2 ounces

Who says you can't eat pancakes and lose weight? Eggs, protein powder, and whole grains turn these pancakes into a powerfully delicious weight-loss ally. Serve them right off the griddle!

Protein: 4 servings protein powder (whey or soy), adjust to your DPR
Protein: 4 eggs plus whites of 2 eggs, adjust to your DPR
2 cups 100% whole-wheat flour
1 tablespoon ground flaxseed
½ cup old-fashioned oats
½ cup unbleached white flour
2 tablespoons baking powder

2 ¼ cups fat-free milk
2 tablespoons olive oil
Nonstick cooking spray

Mix together all the dry ingredients in a large bowl. Mix together the eggs, egg whites, milk, and oil in a separate bowl.

Combine the two mixtures, pouring wet into dry. Use a rubber spatula or spoon to stir from the bottom of the bowl until all the dry ingredients are moistened. *Do not overmix.*

Place a griddle or 12-inch skillet over medium heat. Spray lightly with the nonstick cooking spray. Scoop the batter with a ½-cup measuring cup or spoon and pour onto the hot griddle. Cook the pancakes for 3–4 minutes on the first side, or until the edges begin to dry and bubbles appear in the center of the pancake, then flip to the other side. Flip only once. The remaining pancakes may not take quite as long to cook, as the griddle begins to maintain the heat.

Egg and Spinach Omelet

Prep Time: 5 minutes ▪ Cook Time: 5 minutes ▪ Yield: 1 serving ▪ Protein per Serving Toward DPR: 2 ounces

Experiment by varying the amount of spinach (the more the better), or get creative and toss in other vegetables, too.

Protein: 2 eggs, adjust to your DPR
Nonstick cooking spray
1 ounce low-fat mozzarella cheese, shredded
1 handful (or more) baby spinach
Salsa, unlimited
1 tablespoon fat-free sour cream (optional)

In a small bowl, beat the eggs until fluffy. Spray a small nonstick skillet with cooking spray and heat over medium flame.

Add the eggs and allow to cook until halfway done. When able, use the edge of a spatula to lift the edge of the omelet from the side of the pan and tilt the pan to let the wet egg run underneath the omelet. Continue lifting and tilting until the egg is nearly cooked through.

Add the shredded cheese to one side of the omelet. Add the spinach to the same side of the omelet as the cheese. Using the spatula, lift one side of the omelet and fold it over the cheese and spinach. Cook another 1–2 minutes, until the cheese has melted.

Top with liberal amounts of salsa and, if desired, fat-free sour cream.

Egg and Veggie Scramble

Prep Time: 5 minutes ▪ Cook Time: 5 minutes ▪ Yield: 1 serving ▪ Protein per Serving Toward DPR: 2 ounces

Fresh eggs, baby spinach, and tomatoes ripe off the vine equal yummy protein-packed power! Add more vegetables anytime you like.

Protein: 2 eggs, adjust to your DPR
Nonstick cooking spray
1 handful (or more) baby spinach
1 small tomato, diced
Salsa, unlimited

In a small frying pan coated with the nonstick cooking spray, scramble the eggs over medium heat until nearly cooked through.

Add the baby spinach and continue to cook until the eggs are completely done and the spinach is wilted.

Plate the eggs and top with diced tomatoes. Garnish with spoonfuls of salsa.

Fruit Yogurt Parfait

Prep Time: 5 minutes ▪ Cook Time: 0 minutes ▪ Yield: 1 serving

Enjoy decadent layers of thick yogurt, fruit, and honey. The dry oatmeal adds a European flair.

1½ cups fat-free plain Greek yogurt
Drizzle of honey
½ cup dry old-fashioned oatmeal
Fresh mixed fruit

Start with fruit in the bottom of a parfait or other tall glass, then spoon in yogurt, drizzle of honey, then dry oatmeal. Alternate with layers of fruit, yogurt, honey, and oatmeal, ending with oatmeal.

Garden Veggie Frittata

Prep Time: 20 minutes ▪ Cook Time: 35 minutes ▪ Yield: 6 servings ▪ Protein per Serving Toward DPR: 2 ounces

Elegant enough for brunch with friends, yet simple enough for a weekday morning meal, this frittata affords you time to get ready for your day while it bakes.

Protein: 12 large eggs, adjust to your DPR

1 pound asparagus

6 ounces cremini (brown button) mushrooms

1 tablespoon olive oil

1 clove garlic, minced

1 shallot, finely chopped

1 small zucchini, diced

⅓ cup fat-free milk

1 teaspoon salt

¼ teaspoon freshly ground black pepper

Dash nutmeg

1 tablespoon chopped fresh chives

Nonstick cooking spray

1 large tomato, seeded and thinly sliced

2 tablespoons freshly grated Parmesan cheese

Preheat the oven to 350°F.

Wash and trim the bottom of the asparagus spears and cut on the diagonal into 1-inch pieces. Blanch asparagus in boiling water for 1–2 minutes and immediately plunge into ice water to halt the cooking, then drain; set aside.

Clean and slice the mushrooms. In a skillet, heat the olive oil and sauté the mushrooms over medium heat until they soften, 5–8 minutes. Add the garlic and shallot to the mushrooms and continue to cook for 3–4 minutes more. Remove the mushroom mixture from the heat and set aside.

Slice the zucchini in half lengthwise and then into thin slices.

In a large bowl, beat together the eggs, milk, salt, pepper, nutmeg, and chives. Add the asparagus, mushroom mixture, and zucchini.

Lightly spray a 2-quart baking dish with the nonstick cooking spray. Pour the egg and vegetable mixture into the dish, then arrange the tomatoes on top. Sprinkle the Parmesan cheese over the top.

Bake 30–35 minutes until set.

Mexican Pita with Shrimp

Prep Time: 5 minutes ▪ Cook Time: 5–7 minutes ▪ Yield: 1 serving ▪ Protein per Serving Toward DPR: 2 ounces

When you want something with a little kick in the morning, try this picante pita pocket.

Protein: 2 egg whites, adjust to your DPR
Protein: 4 medium shrimp, precooked, adjust to your DPR
1 whole-wheat pita
1 fresh peach
Nonstick cooking spray
2 ounces low-fat Monterey Jack cheese, shredded
Salsa, unlimited

Cut the pita in half, forming 2 pockets. Toast in a toaster, set aside when done.

Using a sharp knife, score a fresh peach from top to bottom and up the other side. If it's a freestone peach, just twist the two sides in opposite directions and it will come apart cleanly. Carefully remove the pit. In a small nonstick skillet sprayed with cooking spray, place the peach halves cut side down and pan-cook until warmed through and brown on the bottom, 4–5 minutes. Remove the peaches from the pan and set aside.

In the same skillet, add the egg whites and scramble until nearly done, then add the shrimp and cook just until the egg whites are completely done and the shrimp are heated through, 1–2 minutes.

Spoon half the egg mixture into each pita pocket, top with 1 ounce each cheese and ample spoonfuls of salsa. Serve on a small plate with the peaches on the side.

Oat Pudding with Chocolate and Lime

Prep Time: 10–15 minutes ▪ Cook Time: 20 minutes ▪ Yield: 4 servings

Pudding doesn't have to add to your waistline. High fiber with a punch of lime and a sweet hint of chocolate accompany this dish. Serve with a couple of scrambled eggs for a protein boost.

1¼ cups fat-free milk
¾ cup canned light coconut milk
⅓ cup quick-cooking steel-cut oats
2 tablespoons raw brown sugar
2 tablespoons freshly squeezed lime juice
1 ounce 70% or greater fine dark chocolate, grated
¾ teaspoon finely grated lime peel

In a medium saucepan, combine the milk, coconut milk, and oats. Bring to a simmer over medium-high heat and stir occasionally to prevent burning. Reduce the heat to low and simmer, stirring constantly, for 5–8 minutes to yield a thin mixture.

Remove from the heat and stir in the sugar and lime juice. Let stand in the saucepan uncovered until slightly thickened (as long as 10 minutes).

Transfer to ramekins or dessert bowls and garnish with chocolate and lime peel. Serve warm, at room temperature, or chilled.

Overnight Power Oatmeal

Prep Time: 10 minutes ▪ Cook Time: 8-9 hours ▪ Yield: 4 servings ▪ Protein per Serving Toward DPR: about 2 ounces, but depends on brand—check nutrition label

Power up your oatmeal with protein powder for a more satisfying breakfast.

Protein: 1 serving protein powder (Physicians Protein Smoothies Base Mix, or whey, or soy), adjust to your DPR
1 cup steel-cut oats
1 cup dried cranberries
1 cup dried figs
1 piece fresh fruit of your choice (sliced banana, diced apple, peach)
Pinch each of ground cinnamon, cloves, nutmeg, ginger to taste
4 cups water

Combine all ingredients except protein powder in a 2-quart slow cooker. Before bed, cover and set to cook on low heat for 8–9 hours. The following morning, stir, divide into 4 portions, and stir in the protein powder.

If you do not have a slow cooker, use old-fashioned rolled oats instead of steel-cut oats and combine with water in a medium bowl. Cover and refrigerate overnight to allow the oatmeal to "cook." The next morning, reheat the oatmeal over low heat or portion it into 4 small bowls and pop each in the microwave for about 1 minute. Top with protein powder, cranberries, figs, fruit, and spices as desired.

Peanut Butter and Raisin Roll-Up

Prep Time: 10 minutes ▪ Cook Time: 0 minutes ▪ Yield: 1 serving

Feeling like a kid? Go for it with this sophisticated and healthful rendition of a PB&J.

    1 6-inch whole-wheat tortilla
    2 tablespoons natural peanut butter, no sugar added
    2 tablespoons raisins
    ½ banana, sliced

Spread the tortilla with peanut butter. Top with raisins and banana slices and roll it up.

Sausage and Egg Scramble

Prep Time: 5 minutes ▪ Cook Time: 10 minutes ▪ Yield: 4 servings ▪ Protein Per Serving Toward DPR: 2 ounces

This all-American favorite—sausage, eggs, and cheese—gets a mini-makeover.

    Protein: ¼ pound extra lean pork sausage, adjust to your DPR
    Protein: 3 large eggs and whites of 2 eggs, adjust to your DPR
    3 tablespoons fat-free milk
    2 ounces shredded low-fat cheddar cheese
    Salsa, unlimited

If the sausage has a casing, remove it. Then brown the sausage in a medium nonstick skillet until nearly cooked through, breaking it up.

In a smaller bowl, whisk together the eggs, egg whites, and milk and add to the sausage. Stir until the eggs and sausage are cooked through and then top with cheese. Let set for 1–2 minutes to melt the cheese. Top with as much salsa as desired.

Smoked Salmon and Egg Open-Faced Sandwich

Prep Time: 5 minutes ▪ **Cook Time: 5 minutes** ▪ **Yield: 1 serving** ▪ **Protein per Serving Toward DPR: 2 ounces**

Quick and easy, yet elegant and tasty.

    Protein: 2 egg whites, adjust to your DPR
    Protein: 2 slices (1 ounce total) smoked salmon, adjust to your DPR
    Nonstick cooking spray
    ½ small toasted bagel (I like Lender's or Sara Lee)
    2 teaspoons fat-free cream cheese

In a small skillet sprayed with nonstick cooking spray, scramble the egg whites over medium heat. While scrambling the eggs, toast the bagel half and spread with cream cheese. Layer the bagel with scrambled eggs, and top with 2 slices smoked salmon.

Spicy Egg Scramble

Prep Time: 5 minutes ▪ **Cook Time: 10 minutes + set time** ▪ **Yield: 4 servings** ▪ **Protein per Serving Toward DPR: 2 ounces**

Begin your day with this protein powerhouse. Spicing it up helps boost your metabolism.

    Protein: 8 eggs, adjust to your DPR
    3 tablespoons non-trans-fat buttery spread (I like Earth Balance)
    1 tablespoon minced garlic
    1 tablespoon minced ginger
    ½ cup chopped scallions
    1 jalapeño, seeded and minced (use less for less heat)
    Red pepper flakes or pepper sauce to taste (if you want more heat)
    Salt and freshly ground pepper to taste
    ⅓ cup chopped fresh cilantro

Heat the buttery spread over medium-high heat in a nonstick medium skillet. Add the garlic, ginger, scallions, jalapeño, pepper flakes, and salt and pepper. Cook, stirring occasionally, until the garlic begins to brown and the mixture is fragrant, about 3 minutes. Remove from the heat and let cool.

In a medium bowl, beat the eggs, then return the pan to medium-high heat and add in. Stir occasionally, until the eggs are almost done, and remove from the heat.

Mix in the cilantro and serve warm.

Spicy Tofu Scramble

Prep Time: 10 minutes ▪ Cook Time: 15 minutes ▪ Yield: 4 servings ▪ Protein per Serving Toward DPR: 2 ounces

"Piquant" is not a word most would give tofu, but this breakfast cannot be described any other way.

    Protein: 1 pound 8 ounces firm tofu, drained and rinsed, adjust to
        your DPR
    2 tablespoons extra virgin olive oil
    1 cup diced onions
    1 clove garlic, minced
    ½ cup diced red bell pepper
    ½ cup sliced mushrooms
    2 tablespoons white miso paste
    2 tablespoons water
    1½ tablespoons spicy or Dijon mustard
    2 teaspoons curry powder
    ½ tablespoon dried tarragon
    ½ teaspoon chipotle powder
        (or 1 teaspoon chili powder)
    Freshly ground black pepper and salt to taste
    ¼ cup grated soy cheese (optional)

In a large skillet, heat the oil over medium-high heat. Add the onions and sauté until soft, 3–5 minutes. Add the garlic, bell peppers, and mushrooms, and sauté another 5 minutes.

In the meantime, rinse, drain, and crumble the tofu. Add it to the vegetable mixture.

In a small bowl, whisk together the miso and water and pour over the mixture. Stir in the mustard, herbs, and spices and heat through another 5 minutes. Add the cheese, if desired. Cover and let melt.

Zesty Tofu and Spinach Wrap

Prep Time: 5 minutes ■ **Cook Time: 10 minutes** ■ **Yield: 4 servings** ■ **Protein per Serving Toward DPR: 1 ounce**

A tofu wrap is quick and easy, plus it provides ample protein and is rich in calcium.

Protein: 1 12-ounce container extra firm tofu, drained and cut into 1-inch cubes, adjust to your DPR
3 tablespoons extra virgin olive oil
½ medium sweet yellow onion, diced
3 cloves garlic, minced
1 teaspoon lite soy sauce
½ sweet red bell pepper, diced
¾ cup sliced cremini (brown button) mushrooms
2 scallions, sliced
2 tomatoes, seeded and finely chopped
½ teaspoon ground ginger
½ teaspoon chili powder
¼ teaspoon cayenne pepper flakes
6 ounces baby spinach
Salt and freshly ground pepper to taste
4 whole-wheat tortillas or chapattis (Indian flat bread)

Heat the olive oil in a heavy skillet over medium-high heat. Add the onion and garlic and sauté for 4–5 minutes, until the onion begins to soften.

Add the soy sauce, tofu, bell pepper, mushrooms, scallions, tomatoes, ginger, chili powder, and cayenne pepper. Stir frequently and sauté for another 8–10 minutes, until the vegetables are done and the tofu is lightly fried. Add the spinach and sauté until wilted, 1–2 minutes. Add salt and pepper to taste.

Divide the mixture into four servings and spoon onto whole-wheat tortillas or chapattis. Facing the tortilla, fold the bottom half in about 1 inch, then fold in the sides and roll until you have a mini-burrito.

PASTA AND PIZZA

Chicken Pasta with Fresh Summer Vegetables

Prep Time: 15 minutes ▪ Cook Time: 11 minutes ▪ Yield: 6 2-cup servings ▪
Protein per Serving Toward DPR: 4 ounces

Nothing beats freshness like summer vegetables. Be creative in this dish
and mix and match your own favorites.

Protein: 1½ pounds chicken breast, diced, adjust to your DPR
16 ounces whole-grain spaghetti
1 tablespoon olive oil
1 small sweet yellow onion, finely chopped
1 clove garlic, minced
1 yellow bell pepper, thinly sliced
2 small zucchini, diced
2 small yellow squash, diced
1 bunch asparagus, washed and cut into 1-inch pieces
3 cups (1 pint) grape tomatoes, halved
4 fresh basil leaves, torn
Salt and freshly ground black pepper to taste

Cook the spaghetti according to package directions.

Meanwhile, heat the olive oil in a large skillet and sauté the chicken
and onion until the chicken is cooked and the onion begins to soften.
Add the garlic and sauté for 5 minutes. Add the bell pepper, zucchini,
yellow squash, and asparagus, and sauté until heated but not completely cooked (you want the vegetables to have a slight crunch).

Remove from the heat and add the tomatoes, drained spaghetti,
and basil. Season with salt and pepper.

Italian "Sausage" Pizza

Prep Time: 20 minutes ▪ Cook Time: 17 minutes ▪ Yield: 4 servings ▪
Protein per Serving Toward DPR: 4 ounces

Try this chicken "sausage" for a taste sensation that satisfies that sausage
pizza craving.

Protein: 16 ounces boneless skinless chicken breasts, quartered, adjust
   to your DPR
1 10-ounce prepared whole-wheat pizza crust (I like Boboli)
½ teaspoon fennel seeds
¼ yellow sweet onion, halved
1 clove garlic
¼ teaspoon freshly ground black pepper
¼ teaspoon red pepper flakes
Nonstick cooking spray
1 cup pizza sauce
½ cup sliced black olives
5 ounces shredded nonfat mozzarella cheese

Preheat the oven to 450°F. Place the pizza crust on a baking sheet or pizza stone (for extra crunch) and set aside.

In a large dry skillet, over medium-high heat, toast the fennel seeds just until lightly browned, about 1 minute. Using a food processor, pulse the onion and garlic just until minced. Then add the chicken, fennel seeds, and peppers, and pulse until the mixture is ground.

Spray the same large skillet with nonstick cooking spray and brown the chicken mixture over medium heat until cooked through, 7–10 minutes.

Spread the pizza sauce onto the crust. Top with the chicken mixture, olives, and cheese and bake for 7–10 minutes, until the cheese is bubbly and the crust is browned.

Quick and Easy Lemon Pasta

Prep Time: 10 minutes ▪ Cook Time: 20 minutes ▪ Yield: 4 servings

Gruyère has a nutty, slightly sweet taste with complex mushroom notes that balances well with lemon.

1 12-ounce package whole-grain fettuccine noodles
4 medium lemons
½ cup dry white wine
1 cup fat-free sour cream
¾ cup low-fat Gruyère cheese
Salt and freshly ground black pepper to taste

Cook the noodles according to package instructions until al dente and drain (do not rinse). While the pasta is cooking, scrub and dry the lemons then grate them to remove the zest and set aside. Halve the lemons and squeeze the juice from them; remove the seeds.

In a large skillet, boil the wine, lemon juice, and lemon zest until reduced to half the volume. Add the drained pasta to the lemon sauce and toss to coat all the noodles. Stir in the sour cream and grated cheese and simmer until the cream thickens slightly, the cheese is melted, and the pasta is hot. Season to taste with salt and pepper. Garnish with thinly sliced lemons.

Spaghetti and Meat Sauce

Prep Time: 5 minutes ▪ Cook Time: 15–20 minutes ▪ Yield: 4–6 servings ▪ Protein per Serving Toward DPR: 8 ounces

This hearty dish will take you back to your youth. Yummy pasta and meat sauce is comfort food at its best.

    Protein: 2 pounds 95% lean ground beef, adjust to your DPR
1 onion, finely chopped
3 cloves garlic, minced
1 tablespoon olive oil
1 pound whole-wheat spaghetti, broken into thirds
1 16-ounce can stewed tomatoes, cut up
1 14-ounce jar pasta or marinara sauce
1 teaspoon oregano
¼–½ teaspoon crushed red pepper (use more for extra spice)
Salt and freshly ground black pepper to taste

In a large skillet, sauté the onion and garlic in the olive oil over medium-high heat until soft. Add the ground beef and cook, stirring occasionally, until thoroughly cooked.

Meanwhile, cook the spaghetti according to package directions; drain. To the empty spaghetti pot, add the cooked spaghetti, tomatoes, pasta sauce, oregano, red pepper, salt, and pepper. Heat thoroughly over medium heat and enjoy.

Spicy Peanut Noodles

Prep Time: 15 minutes ▪ Cook Time: 30 minutes ▪ Yield: 3 2-cup servings

Plain old pasta gets an exotic Asian twist in this dish that is chock full of fresh, colorful vegetables.

⅓ cup low-fat creamy peanut butter

¼ cup water

2 tablespoons low-sodium soy or tamari sauce

1½ tablespoons rice wine vinegar

1 teaspoon chili paste with garlic (use 2 teaspoons for more spice)

½ teaspoon sugar

8 ounces whole-grain linguine, cooked to package directions

1 medium red bell pepper, cut into thin strips

¾ cup English cucumber, sliced

3 scallions, sliced diagonally into ¼-inch pieces

2 tablespoons chopped cilantro (you can use parsley if you prefer)

6 lime wedges

In a large bowl, combine the peanut butter, water, soy sauce, vinegar, chili paste, and sugar and whisk until blended. The sauce should be creamy and can be thinned with a little water if desired.

Add in the linguine, red bell pepper, cucumber, and scallions, and toss well. Sprinkle with cilantro. Serve with lime wedges.

White Chicken Pizza

Prep Time: 15 minutes ▪ Cook Time: 9 minutes ▪ Yield: 4 servings ▪ Protein per Serving Toward DPR: 4 ounces

Nothing is as satisfying as pizza after a long day at work. Serve with a voluminous side salad and a glass of wine.

Protein: 4 4-ounce chicken breasts, diced, adjust to your DPR

2 shallots, finely diced

4–5 cloves of garlic, minced

Salt and freshly ground pepper to taste

2 tablespoons extra virgin olive oil, divided

1 ball whole-wheat pizza dough (premade and frozen or Boboli)

1 large bunch of fresh basil, finely chopped

1 large handful fresh baby spinach, finely chopped
6-ounces part-skim mozzarella cheese

Preheat the oven to 475°F.

In a medium skillet, sauté the chicken, shallots, garlic, salt, and pepper in 1 tablespoon olive oil over medium heat. When cooked through, remove from the heat and set aside.

Roll out your dough to 12 to 16 inches diameter and brush the top with the remaining olive oil. Spread the chicken mixture evenly across the dough, then add a layer of shredded basil leaves and spinach. Top with shredded cheese and bake for about 9 minutes, until the cheese bubbles and the edges of the crust are golden brown.

SOUPS

Carrot Soup with North African Spices

Prep Time: 15 minutes ▪ Cook Time: 30 minutes ▪ Yield: 4 2-cup servings

The freshness of carrot and ginger partnered with earthy cumin and coriander are a delicious taste duo. Added creaminess comes from the sweet potato.

1 tablespoon olive oil
1 medium yellow onion, thinly sliced
1½ teaspoons salt, divided
4 small garlic cloves, minced
1½ teaspoons cumin seed, toasted and ground
1 teaspoon coriander seed, toasted and ground
3 teaspoons freshly grated ginger or ½ teaspoon dry ginger
1 teaspoon red pepper flakes, toasted and ground (optional)
2 pounds carrots, scrubbed very well and thinly sliced
1 small sweet potato, thinly sliced
5 cups vegetable broth, divided into 4 cups and 1 cup (I like
    low-sodium Frontier)
½ cup freshly squeezed orange juice (squeezed at home or store-bought)
1 teaspoon coarsely chopped cilantro for garnish

Heat the olive oil in a large soup pot or a Dutch oven over medium-high heat and add the onion slices and ½ teaspoon salt. Sauté over medium heat until the onions begin to soften, about 5 minutes, then add the garlic, cumin, coriander, ginger, and red pepper flakes. Cook until the onion is very soft, about 10 more minutes.

Add the carrots, sweet potato, 1 teaspoon salt, and 4 cups vegetable broth. Bring to a gentle boil, then reduce the heat, cover, and simmer until the carrots are very tender, about 15 minutes.

Puree the soup in a blender or food processor until smooth, using extra broth if needed. Return the soup to the pot, and add the orange juice and the last cup of vegetable broth. Garnish each serving with a sprinkle of cilantro.

Hot Black-Eyed Pea Soup

Prep Time: 10 minutes ▪ Cook Time: 40–45 minutes ▪ Yield: 4 1-cup servings ▪ Protein per Serving Toward DPR: 4 ounces

This easy soup is good ol' Southern-style eating. Slow cooker suitable.

Protein: 1 pound cooked boneless chicken breasts, diced, adjust to your DPR
8 ounces dried black-eyed peas
1½–2 cups chicken or vegetable stock
½ cup each, finely chopped celery, onion, carrots, red bell pepper
4–5 cloves garlic, minced
Nonstick cooking spray
1 bay leaf
½ teaspoon salt
Freshly ground black pepper
½ teaspoon red pepper flakes
1 tablespoon seasoning mix (I like Spike)
1 tablespoon fat-free sour cream as garnish (optional)
Unlimited Tabasco or salsa, for topping

Soak the peas in water overnight. In the morning, drain and rinse. In a medium-sized soup pot or Dutch oven over medium heat, bring to a boil the peas and stock. Reduce the heat and simmer 25–30 minutes, until the peas begin to become tender. Add the remaining ingredients, except the sour cream and Tabasco or salsa, and continue to simmer until the vegetables are soft, about 15 minutes.

To prepare in the slow cooker, sauté the celery, onion, carrots, bell pepper, and garlic in a skillet sprayed with nonstick cooking spray over medium heat just until fragrant and beginning to soften, 3–4 minutes.

Remove from the skillet and set aside. Spray with additional cooking spray and quickly sauté the chicken breast until golden on the outside.

Combine everything but the toppings and garnish in the slow cooker, and cook on low 8–9 hours. Top with sour cream and Tabasco or salsa.

Hummus and Pesto Soup

Prep Time: 15 minutes ▪ Cook Time: 10 minutes ▪ Yield: 6 servings

For a high-fiber and filling meal, make this an easy cooking day by using canned beans and vegetable broth powder.

- 3 15-ounce cans chickpeas, drained and rinsed
- 6 cups low-sodium vegetable stock
- 1 small jalapeño, seeded and diced
- 3 tablespoons olive oil
- ¼ cup fresh lemon juice (about 2 lemons)
- 3 tablespoons tahini paste
- 3 small cloves garlic, minced
- 2 teaspoons ground cumin
- 2 teaspoons ground coriander
- 2 teaspoons turmeric
- Salt and freshly ground black pepper to taste
- 6 tablespoons basil or cilantro pesto

If you have a large blender or food processor, blend all the ingredients except the basil or cilantro pesto, and transfer to a large stockpot. If you have a smaller blender or food processor, make this in two batches, blending half the quantity of all the ingredients except the basil or cilantro pesto. Transfer this batch to a large stockpot and repeat with the remaining ingredients until they have all been blended together.

When the soup is mixed together in the pot, bring to a slow boil over medium-high heat, then simmer over low heat, stirring occasionally until heated through.

Ladle the soup into shallow bowls and top with the pesto, which can be swirled in as the soup is eaten. Serve with 2–3 pita chips.

Spinach Garlic Soup

Prep Time: 25 minutes ▪ Cook Time: 10 minutes ▪ Yield: 4 1-cup servings

Pureed soups are an Overnight Diet favorite because they disguise the flavor of vegetables you may think you don't like.

    4 cups chicken or vegetable broth
    ½ cup shredded carrots
    1 10-ounce package fresh spinach, coarsely chopped
    ½ cup chopped onion
    8 cloves garlic, minced
    ¼ cup non-trans-fat buttery spread (I like Earth Balance)
    ¼ cup all-purpose flour
    1 cup fat-free milk
    Salt and freshly ground pepper to taste
    Pinch of ground nutmeg

In a large soup pot or Dutch oven, bring the broth and carrots to a boil over high heat. Reduce the heat and simmer 5 minutes. Stir in the spinach and remove from the heat.

In a small nonstick skillet over medium-high heat, sauté the onion and garlic in the buttery spread until the onion is soft, 5–10 minutes. Add the flour, and stir over low heat for 3–5 minutes until it forms a paste, then slowly add the milk over medium-low heat until a thick and creamy sauce remains. Add this to the broth mixture.

Purée in small batches in a blender or food processor until it reaches the desired consistency. Return the mixture to the soup pot and add the salt, pepper, and nutmeg and heat thoroughly.

Thai Chicken Noodle Soup

Prep Time: 10 minutes ▪ Cook Time: 20 minutes ▪ Yield: 4 1½-cup servings ▪ Protein per Serving Toward DPR: 4 ounces

Soup is always a hit, and this Thai soup has tantalizing aromas of fresh lemongrass. It's the magic potion for a cool evening.

    Protein: 1 pound chicken breasts, cubed, adjust to your DPR
    8–10 ounces dried wide Thai rice noodles

6 cups chicken stock

2 stalks minced lemongrass (or 4 tablespoons prepared lemongrass)

1-inch piece ginger, peeled and minced

2 carrots, sliced

2 cups broccoli florets

2 cups chopped bok choy

½ can light coconut milk

4 tablespoons low-sodium soy sauce

1 tablespoon garlic chili paste, or to taste

Nonstick cooking spray

½ cup roughly chopped fresh basil

Bring a large stockpot of water to a boil and add the noodles. Remove from the heat to allow the noodles to soften while you prepare the broth. In another stockpot over high heat, combine the stock, lemongrass, ginger, and carrots. Bring to a boil, reduce the heat to medium, and simmer while you chop the broccoli and bok choy. Add them to the pot and simmer until the vegetables have softened but are still bright in color, about 5 minutes. Reduce the heat to low and add the coconut milk, soy sauce, and chili paste. In a medium skillet coated with nonstick cooking spray, cook the cubes of chicken until done. Add the chicken to the stockpot.

Drain the noodles and portion out into bowls. Pour several ladles of soup over each bowl of noodles. Sprinkle with fresh basil.

White Bean and Kale Soup

Prep Time: 10 minutes ▪ Cook Time: 7–9 hours ▪ Yield: 9–10 ¾-cup servings

Loaded with antioxidants and filling fiber, kale is at its best when prepared in slow-cooker soups where tenderizing comes from a longer cooking time.

1 large bunch kale

1 ¼ cups small white beans

3 whole garlic cloves, peeled

1 large whole shallot, peeled

3 bay leaves

8 cups vegetable broth (I like low-sodium Frontier)

Freshly ground pepper

1 tablespoon seasoning mix (I like Spike)

Juice of ½ lemon

1 teaspoon salt

1 tablespoon tomato paste

1 teaspoon red pepper flakes

Wash the kale, rinse, and pat dry or spin dry in a salad spinner. Hold each stalk while you pull the leaves off, then discard the stems. Stack the leaves, roll them all together in a bunch, and slice through into ribbons; refrigerate until needed.

Place the white beans, garlic, shallot, bay leaves, vegetable broth, pepper, and seasoning mix in a 3.5-quart slow cooker and cook on high 6–8 hours. (If you don't have a slow cooker, soak the beans overnight, drain, cook until halfway done, then proceed with the recipe. You can also bring them to a rapid boil, cut the heat, cover, and let sit 1 hour.)

An hour before eating, place the kale in a large mixing bowl. Add the lemon juice and salt and scrunch with your hands for 5 minutes to break down the fibers. You'll end up with about one-half the volume.

Add the kale, tomato paste, and pepper flakes to the slow cooker or continue to simmer in a large pot over a low flame and cook another hour or until ready to eat.

POULTRY

Baked Chicken Burritos

Prep Time: 15 minutes ▪ Cook Time: 20 minutes ▪ Yield: 8 servings ▪ Protein per Serving Toward DPR: 4 ounces

These burritos are low-fat and crunchy on the inside with a crispy, flaky outside! This just may become your favorite go-to on busy nights.

Protein: 2 pounds chicken breast strips, adjust to your DPR

1 tablespoon extra virgin olive oil

1 cup chopped onion

1 red bell pepper, chopped

2–3 cloves garlic, crushed

1½ cups canned low-sodium tomato sauce

1 tablespoon chili powder

1–2 teaspoons ground cumin (to taste)

1 teaspoon dried oregano

1 teaspoon dried basil

1 teaspoon salt

½ teaspoon freshly ground black pepper

1 cup frozen whole-kernel corn

¼ cup pitted ripe olives (optional)

¼ cup pine nuts, toasted

¼ cup pumpkin seeds, toasted

Olive oil spray (or other nonstick cooking spray)

8 whole-wheat tortillas or chapattis

½–1 cup grated low-fat Monterey Jack cheese

1 tablespoon guacamole (optional)

1 tablespoon fat-free sour cream (optional)

Unlimited salsa (optional)

Preheat the oven to 350°F. Heat the olive oil in a large nonstick skillet over medium heat, and sauté the chicken, onions, red bell pepper, and garlic until the onion is golden. Add the tomato sauce, chili powder, cumin, oregano, basil, salt, pepper, corn, olives (if using), pine nuts, and pumpkin seeds to the onion mixture, and cook, stirring often, until the mixture begins to boil. Remove from the heat.

Coat a 9-by-13-inch pan lightly with olive oil spray or other nonstick cooking spray. To make a burrito, lay a tortilla down flat, and spread ½ cup of the mixture (or ⅛th of the total amount) over it. Roll, wrapping tightly, and place seam side down in the pan. Repeat until all the tortillas are filled.

Bake the burritos uncovered for 15 minutes or until the tortillas are crisp. Top with grated cheese and bake an additional 5 minutes until melted. Serve the burritos with the toppings of your choice.

Black Bean and Chicken Chili

Prep Time: 10 minutes ▪ Cook Time: 20 minutes ▪ Yield: 4 servings ▪ Protein per Serving Toward DPR: 8 ounces

For more zing, add a few red pepper flakes. For less heat, use fewer jalapeño peppers.

Protein: 2 pounds skinless, boneless chicken breasts, cut into 1-inch pieces, adjust to your DPR

Nonstick cooking spray

1 large red sweet pepper, coarsely diced

1 large sweet yellow onion, chopped

3 tablespoons jalapeño pepper, deseeded and minced

2 cloves garlic, minced

2½ tablespoons flour

2¼ cups fat-free, low-sodium chicken broth

1 15.5-ounce can black beans, drained and rinsed

1 14.5-ounce can diced tomatoes (do not drain)

1 tablespoon ground cumin

½ teaspoon each ground basil, oregano, thyme

2 tablespoons fat-free sour cream

1 large avocado, peeled and diced

Spray a large skillet with nonstick cooking spray. Cook the chicken pieces over medium-high heat until browned, 4–5 minutes, and remove from the heat into a separate dish.

Add more cooking spray to the skillet to sauté the red pepper, onion, jalapeño, and garlic until soft and tender, about 5 minutes, stirring occasionally. Add the flour and stir for 1 minute, until thick, then add the broth, chicken, beans, tomatoes, cumin, basil, oregano, and thyme. Bring to a boil over medium-high heat, then reduce the heat, cover, and simmer until the chicken is cooked through and the vegetables are tender.

Remove from the heat. Stir in the sour cream and garnish with avocado.

Cashew Chicken Salad with Cilantro Dressing

Prep Time: 10 minutes ▪ Cook Time: 5 minutes ▪ Yield: 1 serving ▪ Protein per Serving Toward DPR: 4 ounces

Another quick-cook meal you can whip up in minutes, this filling salad is ideal for lunch or dinner.

Protein: 4 ounces chicken strips, adjust to your DPR

Nonstick cooking spray

⅓ cup sunflower seeds, shelled

1 bunch cilantro, chopped

Juice of 1–2 freshly squeezed oranges

8 ounces mixed lettuces, such as arugula, baby spinach, or mesclun mix
2 tablespoons cashews
1 small tomato, seeded and diced
¼ avocado, sliced
¼ purple onion, sliced thinly
½ cup grated carrots

In a small skillet coated with nonstick cooking spray, sauté the chicken strips over medium heat for 4–6 minutes or until completely cooked through. Remove from the skillet and set aside.

In a small bowl, whisk together the sunflower seeds, chopped cilantro, and freshly squeezed orange juice for the dressing.

In a large mixing bowl, toss together the lettuces, cashews, and cilantro dressing until the lettuces are coated well with dressing.

Plate the lettuces and top with tomato, avocado, purple onion, and carrots.

Chicken and Veggie Stir-Fry

Prep Time: 10 minutes ▪ Cook Time: 15 minutes ▪ Yield: 4 servings ▪ Protein per Serving Toward DPR: 8 ounces

Everybody loves stir-fry, and you'll love how simple it is to make.

Protein: 2 pounds chicken breast, cut into ½-inch cubes, adjust to your DPR
3 tablespoons olive oil
1 pound fresh shiitake mushrooms, sliced
2 tablespoons peeled and minced fresh ginger
3 garlic cloves, minced
2 cups broccoli florets
2 red bell peppers, sliced
2 bunches scallions, sliced
½ cup dry white wine
¼ cup low-sodium soy sauce
1 tablespoon toasted sesame oil
Salt and freshly ground black pepper to taste

Heat 1½ tablespoons olive oil in a large nonstick skillet or wok over high heat. Add the cubed chicken to the hot oil, and sauté until no longer pink. Stir gently until it begins to brown around the edges, about 4 minutes.

While the chicken cooks, remove the stems from the mushrooms and slice the caps. Prepare the broccoli and slice the scallions.

When done, remove the chicken from the heat to a bowl. Add 1½ tablespoons oil, the ginger, and the garlic to the skillet; stir 1 minute. Add the mushrooms; stir-fry until tender, about 5 minutes. Add the broccoli, bell peppers, and scallions; stir-fry until the vegetables are crisp-tender, about 3 minutes. Return the chicken to the skillet and stir to mix in with the vegetables. Stir together the white wine, soy sauce, and sesame oil in a separate bowl and add to the chicken mixture. Heat through for 1 minute. Season with salt and pepper, if desired.

Extra-Healthy Spinach Salad with Turkey

Prep Time: 10 minutes ▪ Cook Time: 20 minutes ▪ Yield: 8 servings ▪ Protein per Serving Toward DPR: 4 ounces

This voluminous salad is tasty enough to please the entire family.

Protein: 2 pounds turkey breast, cubed, adjust to your DPR
1 large egg
¼ cup unbleached white flour
3 teaspoons garlic powder
1 teaspoon onion powder
½ teaspoon freshly ground black pepper
3 tablespoons + ½ cup extra virgin olive oil
½ cup white wine vinegar
¼ cup sugar
3 tablespoons orange juice
3 ounces baby spinach
3 ounces mesclun mix
1 15-ounce can mandarin oranges, drained
½ cup chopped walnuts
½ cup dried cranberries
1 red bell pepper, sliced
½ cup feta cheese (optional)

Beat the egg in a small bowl. In another small bowl, mix together the flour, garlic and onion powders, and black pepper. Dip the turkey cubes in the egg, and dust with the flour mixture.

Heat 3 tablespoons oil in a large skillet over medium-high heat. Sauté the turkey cubes about 10 minutes, turning them so they are golden and crispy on all sides. Remove from the pan and allow to cool. In a small saucepan, combine ½ cup olive oil, white wine vinegar, sugar, and orange juice and cook over medium heat 2–3 minutes, until the sugar dissolves. Transfer to a bowl and allow to cool.

Rinse and dry the spinach and mesclun mix, and place them in a large serving bowl. Add the mandarin oranges, walnuts, cranberries, and red bell pepper. Add half of the dressing, toss well, and plate in 8 individual salad bowls. Garnish with turkey cubes and feta cheese (if using) and drizzle remaining salad dressing evenly over all the plates.

Healthy Layered Vegetable Salad with Bacon

Prep Time: 20 minutes ▪ Cook Time: 8 minutes; Chill Time: 2–4 hours ▪ Yield: 5 2-cup servings ▪ Protein per Serving Toward DPR: ¼ ounce

This version of the potluck and picnic favorite boasts all the flavor without all the extra fat and calories.

Protein: 5 slices low-fat turkey bacon, cooked to a crisp then crumbled (I like Oscar Mayer Louis Rich), adjust to your DPR

6 cups salad greens (red-tipped lettuce is soft and sweet and adds color)

2 cups broccoli florets

1 cup shredded carrots

2 cups frozen green peas, thawed

1 medium red or orange bell pepper, thinly sliced

1–2 stalks celery, thinly sliced

½ cup scallions (green part), thinly sliced

¾ cup fat-free mayonnaise

¾ cup low-fat buttermilk

½ teaspoon dried basil leaves (feel free to experiment with other herbs)

Zest of 1 lemon

1 teaspoon freshly squeezed lemon juice

Salt and freshly ground black pepper to taste
½ cup 50% or 75% reduced-fat Cheddar cheese

Cook the bacon according to package directions, about 8 minutes. Remove to a paper towel to drain and cool. Crumble.

Place the salad greens in a large glass serving bowl. Layer the broccoli, carrots, peas, pepper, celery, and bacon, ending with the scallions on top.

In a small bowl, whisk together the mayonnaise, buttermilk, basil, lemon zest, lemon juice, and salt and pepper for the dressing. Pour the dressing over the salad and sprinkle with the cheese.

Cover with plastic wrap and chill in the refrigerator for 2–4 hours. Toss well before serving.

Indian Spiced Chicken

Prep Time: 10 minutes ▪ **Cook Time: 20 minutes** ▪ **Yield: 2 servings** ▪ **Protein per Serving Toward DPR: 8 ounces**

Curry, cumin, coriander, mint, turmeric, and ginger—these zesty spices give chicken an exotic flair.

Protein: 2 8-ounce boneless chicken breasts, adjust to your DPR
1 teaspoon curry powder
½ teaspoon salt
½ teaspoon crushed red pepper
1 teaspoon ground cumin
1 teaspoon ground coriander
1 teaspoon dried mint
½ teaspoon turmeric
½ teaspoon ground ginger
Nonstick cooking spray

Preheat the oven to 350°F. Mix together the curry powder, salt, crushed red pepper, cumin, coriander, mint, turmeric, and ginger in a small bowl.

Wash the chicken breasts in water and pat dry. Spray each side of the chicken with nonstick cooking spray, then sprinkle with the spice mix. Bake for 15–20 minutes until the chicken is no longer pink.

Shepherd's Pie with Chicken

Prep Time: 20 minutes ■ Cook Time: 1 hour ■ Yield: 8 servings ■ Protein per Serving Toward DPR: 2 ounces

If you like potpie, you're in for a real treat with this 6-Day Fuel Up–friendly version.

FILLING

Protein: 1 pound chicken breast, cubed, adjust to your DPR
1 sweet yellow onion, thinly sliced
½ cup green beans, cut into 1-inch pieces
½ cup zucchini, halved lengthwise and sliced
1 large carrot, sliced and peeled
1 large parsnip, sliced and peeled
½ cup frozen peas, thawed
1 cup mushrooms, sliced

MASHED POTATOES

4 large Yukon gold or russet potatoes
3 tablespoons non-trans-fat buttery spread (I like Earth Balance)
½ teaspoon no-salt onion powder
½ teaspoon coarsely ground black pepper

GRAVY

¼ cup whole-wheat flour
1½ cups hot vegetable broth (I like low-sodium Frontier)
2 tablespoons tamari
2 tablespoons nutritional yeast (*not* baker's or brewer's yeast) (I like Red Star or Bragg)
Salt and freshly ground black pepper to taste

Preheat the oven to 375°F. In a medium skillet over medium-high heat, sauté the chicken cubes until they are cooked through; set aside.

Scrub and cube the unpeeled potatoes. In a large stockpot, bring 4 quarts of water to a boil over high heat then reduce the heat to a soft boil and cook until tender, about 20 minutes. Drain and mash, then add the buttery spread, onion powder, and pepper. While the potatoes are cooking, prepare the vegetables and steam them just until they are beginning to soften, about 5 minutes.

In a heavy skillet over medium heat, heat the flour and continuously stir with a wooden spoon until it becomes a rich brown color. Very slowly add the hot vegetable broth and tamari, stirring constantly to avoid lumps, until completely dissolved and heated, about 5 minutes. Stir in the nutritional yeast, salt, and pepper. Mix in the chicken and vegetables and place in a 3-quart casserole dish. Cover with mashed potatoes and bake for 40 minutes, until golden brown.

Spicy Chicken and White Bean Chili

Prep Time: 20 minutes ▪ Cook Time: 20 minutes ▪ Yield: 4 1½-cup servings ▪ Protein per Serving Toward DPR: 4 ounces

High in both protein and fiber, this spicy chili will keep you going for hours.

Protein: 1 pound skinless, boneless chicken breast, cut into 1-inch pieces, adjust to your DPR

Nonstick cooking spray

1 large onion, chopped

1 medium jalapeño pepper, seeded and minced

2–3 cloves garlic, minced

3 tablespoons unbleached white flour

2½ cups low-sodium, fat-free chicken broth

1 19-ounce can cannellini beans, rinsed and drained

1 tablespoon ground cumin

Pinch of red pepper flakes or cayenne pepper

2 tablespoons fat-free sour cream

Juice of 1 lime

1 medium avocado, sliced

2 tablespoons salsa (optional)

Spray a large skillet with nonstick cooking spray. Sauté the chicken pieces over medium-high heat until brown, about 5 minutes. Remove to a plate.

Spray the same skillet with additional cooking spray and sauté the onion, jalapeño, and garlic over medium-high heat until tender. Add the flour, stirring quickly, and cook for 1 minute. Stir in the broth, chicken, beans, cumin, and red pepper flakes. Bring to a boil over high heat. Reduce the heat to low and simmer until the chicken is no longer pink and the vegetables are tender, about 10 minutes. Remove from the heat.

Stir in the sour cream first and then add the lime juice. Spoon into 4 serving bowls and top each bowl with one-quarter of the avocado slices. Add salsa, if desired.

Thai Chicken Salad

Prep Time: 10 minutes ▪ Cook Time: 0 minutes ▪ Yield: 4 servings ▪ Protein per Serving Toward DPR: 4 ounces

No cooking required for this protein-rich Thai sensation!

    Protein: 1 pound precooked chicken breasts, cut into 1-inch pieces,
        adjust to your DPR
    4 cups chopped lettuce greens
    1 cup diced unpeeled English cucumber
    1 cup tomato, seeded and diced
    ½ cup sliced scallions
    1 cup low-sodium, fat-free chicken broth
    2 tablespoons smooth natural peanut butter,
        no sugar added
    1 tablespoon low-sodium soy sauce
    1 teaspoon lime zest
    2 tablespoons freshly squeezed lime juice
    2 teaspoons toasted sesame oil
    ¼ cup chopped dry roasted peanuts

Divide the lettuce onto 4 individual plates. Top with the chicken, cucumber, tomato, and scallions.

To make the dressing, whisk together in a small bowl the broth, peanut butter, soy sauce, lime zest and juice, and toasted sesame oil. Drizzle the dressing over the salad. Top with peanuts.

Zesty Broccoli Slaw Salad with Chicken

Prep Time: 15–20 minutes ▪ Cook Time: 0 ▪ Yield: 4 servings ▪ Protein per Serving Toward DPR: 8 ounces

Another no-cook meal! Just toss it all together for a super easy, tasty dish.

> Protein: 2 pounds precooked chicken tenders, adjust to
> your DPR
> 1 1-pound package broccoli slaw
> 1 small red bell pepper, thinly sliced
> ⅓ cup chopped cilantro
> 2 scallions, chopped
> 4 tablespoons chopped roasted peanuts
> 2 tablespoons toasted sesame oil
> 1 tablespoon rice vinegar
> 1 tablespoon balsamic vinegar
> 1 teaspoon Sriracha or other chili-garlic sauce
> 1 teaspoon agave nectar

In a large bowl, combine the chicken, broccoli slaw, red pepper, cilantro, and scallions. In a small bowl, whisk together the sesame oil, vinegars, Sriracha sauce, and agave nectar. Pour the dressing over the salad, and toss. Top with chopped peanuts.

BEEF AND PORK

Beefy Mushroom Burgers

Prep Time: 15 minutes ▪ Cook Time: 16–20 minutes ▪ Yield: 4 servings ▪ Protein per Serving Toward DPR: 4 ounces

Yes! You can eat a hamburger and still lose weight, if you make it the Overnight Diet way.

> Protein: 1 pound 90% lean ground beef, adjust to
> your DPR
> 1 ounce dried mushrooms (porcini, shiitake, or
> cremini)

Salt and freshly ground black pepper to taste
2 teaspoons Worcestershire sauce
½ pound fresh button, cremini, or shiitake mushrooms, sliced
1 large sweet yellow onion, thinly sliced
2 tablespoon olive oil
4 light whole-wheat burger buns
Lettuce, tomatoes, and pickles (optional)

Pulse the dried mushrooms in a food processor. In a large bowl, thoroughly mix together the processed mushrooms, ground beef, salt, pepper, and Worcestershire sauce (use your hands to get a better mixture). Shape the meat into 4 patties, and using your thumb, make an indentation in the center of each burger.

Prepare your grill on high heat. While the grill is warming up, heat a large heavy sauté pan over high heat for 1 minute. Add the fresh mushrooms and dry-sauté them until they release their water, 2–3 minutes. Add the onions and the olive oil, toss to combine, and continue to sauté over high heat 1 minute. Add salt to taste and cook until the onions soften and begin to brown. Turn off the heat and place in a bowl.

Grill the burgers to desired doneness, between 5 and 8 minutes per side. Place a grilled burger on the bottom layer of the bun, then top with sautéed mushrooms and onions. Add lettuce, tomatoes, and pickles, if desired.

Braised Tenderloin Cutlets in Mushroom and Red Wine Sauce

Prep Time: 15 minutes ▪ Cook Time: 12–18 minutes ▪ Yield: 2 servings ▪ Protein per Serving Toward DPR: 8 ounces

Steak and mushrooms are another all-American favorite. Try them with quinoa and a large side salad for a twist.

Protein: 2 8-ounce tenderloin steaks, adjust to your DPR
1 tablespoon + 1 teaspoon unbleached flour
1 tablespoon olive oil
¼ pound cremini (brown button) mushrooms, sliced
¼ cup finely chopped sweet yellow onion

2 cloves garlic, minced

½ cup dry red wine

1 teaspoon Dijon or spicy brown mustard

½ teaspoon dried thyme

½ cup vegetable broth (I like low-sodium Frontier)

¼ cup chopped parsley

Coat the tenderloin steak pieces in 1 tablespoon flour. Heat the oil in a large Dutch oven or large pot over medium-high heat. Add the tenderloin when the oil is hot, and cook 1–2 minutes on each side. Remove the steak from the pot and cover to keep warm.

Add the mushrooms, onion, and garlic to the pot. Sauté 7–10 minutes or until softened and lightly browned. Whisk together the red wine, mustard, and thyme in a measuring cup. Add to the mushroom mixture. Season with salt and pepper, if desired, and cook another 2–3 minutes, until the sauce is slightly thickened. Whisk together 1 teaspoon flour and the vegetable broth, then add to the mushroom mixture. Simmer 2–3 minutes or until thickened, stirring constantly.

Plate the steak cutlets and top with the mushroom sauce. Add a sprinkle of parsley.

Fiery Barbecue Pulled Pork

Prep Time: 20–30 minutes ▪ Cook Time: 4½ hours ▪ Yield: 4 servings ▪ Protein per Serving Toward DPR: 8 ounces

Spicy and tangy barbecue is reminiscent of sizzling summer days. Pair it with fresh vegetable sides such as vinegary coleslaw or a chopped salad.

Protein: 2 pounds boneless pork ribs, adjust to your DPR

1 14-ounce can low-sodium beef broth

1 18-ounce bottle barbecue sauce

1 tablespoon spicy chili paste

½ teaspoon liquid smoke

4 whole-wheat light burger buns

Place the ribs into a slow cooker and pour in the beef broth. Cook on high heat for 4 hours, until the meat is very tender. If you don't have a slow cooker, bring the beef and broth to a boil in a large pot.

Then reduce the heat to low-medium, add the ribs, and simmer until very tender. Remove the meat and shred with two forks.

Preheat the oven to 350°F. Add the shredded pork to a cast iron skillet (or Dutch oven) and stir in the barbecue sauce, chili paste, and liquid smoke. Bake in the preheated oven for 30 minutes.

Remove from the oven and divide between 4 burger buns.

Meatloaf

Prep Time: 15 minutes ▪ Cook Time: 60 minutes ▪ Yield: 6 slices ▪ Protein per Serving Toward DPR: 4 ounces

Who knew meatloaf could be low in fat, high in fiber, and so delicious? Cold meatloaf sandwiches on whole-grain bread make an excellent lazy day lunch the next day.

Protein: 1½ pounds 95% lean ground beef, adjust to your DPR
Nonstick cooking spray
1 medium onion, diced
1 stalk celery, sliced
1 red bell pepper, diced
3 cloves garlic, minced
3 tablespoons extra virgin olive oil
¼ cup finely chopped walnuts
¼ cup quick-cooking oats, uncooked
1 slice whole-wheat bread, crumbled
¼ cup ketchup or barbecue sauce
¼ cup brown sugar
½ teaspoon dry mustard
½ teaspoon nutmeg
Salt and freshly ground black pepper to taste

Preheat the oven to 375°F. Spray a 9-by-5-by-3-inch loaf pan with nonstick cooking spray. In a large skillet, sauté the ground beef, onion, celery, red bell peppers, and garlic in olive oil until the onions are soft and translucent.

In a large bowl, combine the mixture with the walnuts, oats, bread crumbles, ketchup or barbecue sauce, brown sugar, and seasonings. Using your hands, mix well, then press into the loaf pan.

Add a little extra water if the texture seems too dry. Cover with foil and bake for 30 minutes. Uncover and bake another 5 minutes until the top is browned.

Old-Fashioned Beef Stew

Prep Time: 30 minutes ▪ Cook Time: 1 hour, 30 minutes ▪ Yield: 12 servings ▪ Protein per Serving Toward DPR: 8 ounces

This hearty beef stew is reminiscent of Sundays past. Pair it with a colorful salad to meet all your nutrient needs.

Protein: 6 pounds boneless chuck roast, cut into 2-inch pieces (or stew beef), adjust to your DPR

3 tablespoons olive oil

2 teaspoons salt

1 tablespoon freshly ground pepper

2 yellow onions, quartered

¼ cup unbleached white flour

3 cloves garlic, minced

1 cup dry red wine

3 cups fat-free beef broth

½ teaspoon dried rosemary

1 bay leaf

½ teaspoon dried thyme

1 large russet potato, unpeeled, scrubbed, and cut into small cubes

6 carrots, unpeeled, scrubbed, and sliced into ½-inch slices

2 stalks celery, sliced into ½-inch slices

Fresh parsley (optional)

Heat the olive oil in a large, heavy-bottomed Dutch oven or stockpot over medium-high heat. When the oil is hot, add the beef and brown well on all sides. Once browned, add the salt and pepper and remove the beef with a slotted spoon. Set aside.

Add the onions and sauté for about 5 minutes, until softened. Reduce the heat to medium-low, add the flour, and cook for 2 minutes, stirring often until thick. Add the garlic and cook for 1 minute. Pour in the wine to deglaze the pan, scraping any brown bits stuck to the bottom of the pan with a spatula. The flour will start to thicken the wine as it comes to a simmer. Simmer another 5 minutes, and then add the broth, rosemary, bay leaf, thyme, and beef. Bring back to a gentle simmer, cover, and cook on very low for about 1 hour.

Add the potatoes, carrots, and celery, and simmer covered for another 30 minutes or until the meat and vegetables are tender.

Allow to sit for another 15 minutes off the heat and covered tightly. Garnish with the fresh parsley if desired.

Rosemary Pork Roast

Prep Time: 10 minutes ▪ Cook Time: 2 hours ▪ Yield: 6 servings ▪ Protein per Serving Toward DPR: 8 ounces

Pork roast doesn't have to be complicated to cook—this one is fast, simple, and succulent. You won't be disappointed.

  Protein: 3 pounds pork tenderloin, adjust to your DPR
  1 tablespoon + 2 teaspoons olive oil
  4–8 cloves garlic, halved
  3 tablespoons dried rosemary, chopped

Preheat the oven to 375°F. Pour 1 tablespoon olive oil into a large, heavy Dutch oven or stockpot with a lid and add the tenderloin. Rub the tenderloin liberally with 2 teaspoons olive oil, then lay the garlic halves on top of it. Sprinkle with the rosemary.

Bake with the lid on for 2 hours, or until the internal temperature of the pork reaches 160°F.

If using a slow cooker instead of baking, add 1–2 cups of water (so the water reaches at least 1 inch of the roast). Cover and cook on low heat 8–9 hours, until roast is tender and pulls apart with a fork.

Vegetable Stir-Fry (with Beef or Pork)

Prep Time: 5–8 minutes ▪ Cook Time: 8–10 minutes ▪ Yield: 4 servings ▪ Protein per Serving Toward DPR: 4 ounces

Broccoli, cauliflower, sugar snap peas, and carrots add sparkles of dazzling color and calcium to boot. Add in flavorful beef or pork to round out the meal.

  Protein: 1 pound lean beef or pork, cut into cubes, adjust to your DPR
  2 cloves garlic, minced

1-inch piece ginger, peeled and minced
2 tablespoons hoisin sauce
2 cups cauliflower florets
1 cup sugar snap peas
1 large carrot, sliced
1 medium onion, thinly sliced
2 cups broccoli florets
1 tablespoon extra virgin olive oil
2 tablespoons water
3 tablespoons dry cooking sherry or rice wine vinegar
1½ teaspoons cornstarch dissolved in ½ cup cold water

Combine the garlic, ginger, and hoisin sauce in a small bowl and set aside.

Prepare the vegetables by cutting them into small, bite-sized pieces. Heat the oil in a large heavy-bottomed skillet (with a lid) over medium-high heat and sauté the beef or pork until nearly done. Add the cauliflower, sugar snap peas, carrot, and onion. Stir-fry for 4–5 minutes, then add the broccoli and water, cover, and cook for another 4–5 minutes, until the vegetables are still crisp but tender.

Add the ginger sauce, sherry, and the cornstarch mixture, and stir until the sauce is thickened.

SEAFOOD

Apple Tuna Roll-Up

Prep Time: 2–4 minutes ▪ Cook Time: 5–6 minutes ▪ Yield: 3 servings ▪ Protein per Serving Toward DPR: 4 ounces

This recipe takes the typical tuna sandwich in a tasty new healthful direction.

Protein: 2 6 ½-ounce cans chunk light tuna in water, drained, adjust to your DPR
¼ cup fat-free plain Greek yogurt
1 small apple, cored and chopped
1 teaspoon mustard (Dijon, spicy brown, yellow)

1 teaspoon honey or agave nectar

3 whole-wheat lavash (I like Joseph's Flax, Oat Bran & Whole Wheat Square Lavash)

1½ cups lettuce greens (mesclun mix, baby spinach, romaine, spring mix)

1 medium tomato, seeded and diced

1 large carrot, grated

1 medium fresh beet, grated (I like to use yellow whenever possible)

1 cup alfalfa sprouts (or sunflower shoots)

1 cup red grapes

In a small bowl, mix together the tuna, yogurt, apple, mustard, and honey. Spread evenly on each lavash. Top with lettuce, tomato, grated carrot, grated beet, and sprouts. Cut each lavash in half and serve with a side of red grapes.

Crusty Oven-Fried Fish

Prep Time: 10 minutes ▪ Cook Time: 8 minutes ▪ Yield: 4 servings ▪ Protein per Serving Toward DPR: 8 ounces

Love fish but not sure how to cook it? This oven-fried fish is as easy as it gets.

Protein: 4 8-ounce pieces cod (¾–1-inch thick), adjust to your DPR

¾ cup plain dried bread crumbs

¾ cup yellow cornmeal

2 tablespoons finely grated Parmesan cheese

1 teaspoon salt

¼ teaspoon black pepper

¼ teaspoon cayenne pepper

1 egg and 2 egg whites, lightly beaten

3 tablespoons olive oil

Preheat the oven to 500°F. Combine the bread crumbs, cornmeal, Parmesan cheese, salt, pepper, and cayenne pepper in a large plastic bag that has a zippered seal. Shake to thoroughly mix.

Place the fish into the plastic bag one at a time to coat. Then dip the fish into the slightly beaten egg mixture and drop into the plastic bag for a second coat of crumb mixture.

Line a baking sheet with parchment paper or aluminum foil. Spread the olive oil onto the paper or foil. Add the fish to the pan and cook in the oven about 4 minutes, then flip the fish over to the other side for another 4 minutes, until both sides are golden brown and the fish is flaky when pierced with a fork.

Lemon Roasted Salmon

Prep Time: 15 minutes ▪ **Cook Time: 15 minutes** ▪ **Yield: 4 servings** ▪
Protein per Serving Toward DPR: 8 ounces

Select wild salmon over farm raised for a mild, "not so fishy" flavor.

 Protein: 4 8-ounce salmon fillets, adjust to your DPR
 1 teaspoon grated lemon zest
 2 tablespoons fresh lemon juice
 2 tablespoons honey
 ½ teaspoon salt
 ½ teaspoon ground coriander seeds
 ¼ teaspoon ground cayenne pepper
 1 6-ounce can thawed orange juice concentrate
 Nonstick cooking spray
 1 small orange, sliced thin

Preheat the oven to 400°F. Whisk together the lemon zest, lemon juice, honey, salt, coriander, cayenne pepper, and orange juice concentrate in a bowl. Place the fish skin side down in a large casserole pan and pour the citrus mixture on top. Let set for 10 minutes. Transfer the fish to a thick baking pan coated with cooking spray. Bake for 15 minutes or until the fish flakes easily with a fork. Garnish with the orange slices.

Magician Salad with Ahi Tuna

Prep Time: 15 minutes ▪ **Cook Time: 5–6 minutes** ▪ **Yield: 2 servings** ▪
Protein per Serving Toward DPR: 4 ounces

The sesame miso dressing almost magically takes an ordinary salad and turns it into an extraordinary Asian-infused creation.

 Protein: 2 4-ounce wild ahi tuna steaks, adjust to your DPR
 6 cups mesclun lettuce
 ½ cup shredded carrots
 ½ cup sunflower sprouts

⅓ cup rice wine vinegar
¼ cup white miso paste
2 tablespoons freshly squeezed lemon juice
2 teaspoons grated ginger
1 tablespoon organic sugar
2 tablespoons toasted sesame seeds + seeds to garnish
1 teaspoon toasted sesame oil
3 tablespoons mirin or cooking sake

In a medium-sized cast iron or thick-bottomed skillet, pan sear the tuna over medium-high heat for 1–2 minutes on each side; the tuna will still be uncooked in the middle. If desired, cook the tuna until well done, 3–4 minutes per side.

In a medium-sized mixing bowl, toss together the mesclun lettuce, carrots, and sprouts. In a separate smaller bowl, whisk together the vinegar, miso, lemon juice, ginger, sugar, sesame seeds, sesame oil, and mirin. Drizzle over the lettuce mixture and toss well to coat.

Portion the salad into 2 large servings; top with tuna steak. Garnish with a few sesame seeds.

Mediterranean Tuna Salad

Prep Time: 10–12 minutes ▪ Cook Time: 0 minutes ▪ Yield: 4 servings ▪ Protein per Serving Toward DPR: 4 ounces

Chickpeas, also known as garbanzo beans, are a fiber- and protein-rich addition. Add colorful vegetables for an antioxidant boost.

    Protein: 3 5-ounce cans water-packed chunk light tuna, drained well, adjust to your DPR
    Protein: 2 hard-boiled egg whites, finely diced, adjust to your DPR
    ½ 15-ounce can chickpeas, rinsed and drained
    1 large red bell pepper, finely diced
    ½ cup finely chopped red onion
    ½ cup chopped fresh parsley
    4 teaspoons capers, rinsed
    1½ teaspoons finely chopped fresh rosemary

½ cup lemon juice, divided in half

4 tablespoons extra virgin olive oil, divided in half

Freshly ground black pepper to taste

¼ teaspoon salt

8 cups mixed salad greens (such as mesclun mix, baby spinach, and arugula)

Combine the tuna, egg whites, chickpeas, bell pepper, onion, parsley, capers, rosemary, ¼ cup lemon juice, and 2 tablespoons oil in a medium bowl. Combine the pepper and remaining ¼ cup lemon juice, 2 tablespoons oil, and salt in a separate large bowl. Add the salad greens and toss to coat. Divide the greens among 4 plates. Top each with one-fourth of the tuna salad.

Pan-Fried Wild Salmon and Mustard Sauce

Prep Time: 10 minutes ▪ Cook Time: 20 minutes ▪ Yield: 4 servings ▪ Protein per Serving Toward DPR: 8 ounces

Take a walk on the wild side with spicy wild salmon fillets.

Protein: 4 8-ounce wild salmon fillets, 1-inch thick, adjust to your DPR

1 tablespoon olive oil

Freshly ground black pepper

½ cup vegetable broth (I like low-sodium Frontier)

2 tablespoons balsamic vinegar

1 tablespoon Dijon or spicy brown mustard

2 teaspoons packed dark brown sugar

Heat the oil in a medium skillet over medium heat. Coat the flesh side of the salmon with pepper. Place the salmon, skin side up, into the hot skillet, and cook for about 4 minutes on each side, until cooked through. (If preferred, cook less so it remains slightly under-cooked in the middle.) Remove the salmon to a plate; cover to keep warm and set aside.

To the skillet, add the broth, balsamic vinegar, mustard, and brown sugar. Heat to a boil. Cook over medium heat until the mixture is slightly thickened and reduced to ¼ cup, about 10 minutes. Serve over the salmon.

Spicy Tuna Delight

Prep Time: 10 minutes ▪ Cook Time: 0 minutes ▪ Yield: 4 servings ▪ Protein per Serving Toward DPR: 4 ounces

This tuna salad has a zesty zing. Use mild salsa to tone down the heat; extra spicy salsa for more heat—it's all up to you.

Protein: 3 5-ounce cans chunk light tuna in water, drained, adjust to your DPR

Protein: 2 hard-boiled egg whites, diced, adjust to your DPR

½ cup sliced ripe black olives

½ cup sliced scallions

½ cup thinly sliced celery

⅔ cup salsa

½ cup fat-free sour cream

1 teaspoon ground cumin

Lettuce leaves, shredded

Raw vegetables for serving (such as cauliflower or broccoli florets, red bell pepper, carrot or celery sticks, raw zucchini slices)

In a medium bowl, combine the tuna, egg whites, olives, scallions, and celery. In a separate small bowl, blend together the salsa, sour cream, and cumin, and pour over the tuna mixture. Stir until the tuna mixture is evenly coated with the salsa.

To serve, fill 4 serving plates with shredded lettuce. Top with one-fourth of the tuna mixture and surround with cut vegetables. Drizzle with extra salsa, if desired.

VEGETABLES, SNACKS, AND SIDE DISHES

Apples with Creamy Peanut Dip

Prep Time: 10 minutes ▪ Cook Time: 0 minutes ▪ Yield: 4 servings

Dip apples into creamy peanut velvet for a filling snack.

8 ounces fat-free cream cheese, softened

2 tablespoons light brown sugar

1½ teaspoons vanilla or almond extract

2 teaspoons orange juice (fresh-squeezed or store-bought)

2 tablespoons coarsely chopped peanuts

4 apples, cored, seeded, and sliced

Combine the cream cheese, brown sugar, extract, and orange juice in a small bowl and mix until smooth. Stir in the chopped peanuts.

Dip apples slices and enjoy!

Avocado, Fennel, and Citrus Salad

Prep Time: 20 minutes ▪ Cook Time: 0 minutes ▪ Yield: 4 servings

Light and refreshing, this salad can be paired with beef, poultry, or seafood dishes.

1 orange

1 ruby red grapefruit

3 tablespoons white balsamic or red wine vinegar

2 teaspoons fennel seeds, toasted and crushed

3 tablespoons olive oil

Salt and pepper to taste

2 large ripe avocados, peeled and halved

1 fennel bulb, cut in half, thinly sliced

1 cup pea sprouts, or sunflower sprouts

2 tablespoons finely chopped shallot

Grate ¼ teaspoon zest from the orange. Peel the orange and grapefruit and, using a small, sharp knife, cut the juicy sections away from the white membranes. Work over a small bowl to catch any juice.

In the same bowl, whisk together the vinegar, fennel seeds, orange zest, and 1 tablespoon orange juice and 1 tablespoon grapefruit juice caught from each fruit for the salad dressing. Gradually whisk in the oil. Add salt and freshly ground pepper to taste.

On each serving plate, place an avocado half and drizzle 1 teaspoon of the dressing over each. Toss sliced fennel, sprouts, and shallots with enough remaining dressing to coat. Generously top the avocado halves with the fennel mixture and allow it to overflow the avocado. Arrange reserved grapefruit and orange segments around the avocados. Drizzle more of the remaining dressing over the fennel and orange and grapefruit segments.

Baked Cinnamon Apples

Prep Time: 5 minutes ▪ Cook Time: 30–40 minutes ▪ Yield: 4 servings

When you're craving a sweet snack, reach for these delectably spiced baked apples.

    4 baking apples (Honeycrisp, Golden Delicious, Jonathon, Melrose, or
       Winesap)
    4 tablespoons packed dark brown sugar
    4 teaspoons non-trans-fat buttery spread (I like Earth Balance)
    ½ teaspoon ground cinnamon
    ¼ teaspoon ground cloves
    ¼ cup water

Preheat the oven to 375°F. Core the apples and set upright in an 8-by-8-inch glass baking dish. In the center of each apple, place 1 tablespoon sugar, 1 teaspoon buttery spread, and a pinch of cinnamon and cloves (or more if you like a spicier taste). Pour the water into the pan and bake for 30–40 minutes, until the apples are soft.

Baked Parmesan Tomatoes

Prep Time: 2–4 minutes ▪ Cook Time: 15 minutes ▪ Yield: 4 servings

Crispy on top, soft and juicy on the bottom, baked tomatoes serve as an impeccable complement to any dinner. In the summertime, choose heirloom tomatoes for their authentic colors and unbeatable taste.

    4 tomatoes, halved horizontally
    ⅓ cup grated low-fat Parmesan cheese
    1 teaspoon chopped fresh oregano
    Pinch of salt to taste
    Freshly ground black pepper to taste
    4 teaspoons extra virgin olive oil

Preheat the oven to 450° F. Place the tomatoes cut side up on a baking sheet. Top with the Parmesan, oregano, salt, and pepper. Drizzle with oil and bake until the tomatoes are tender, about 15 minutes.

Berry, Jicama, and Apple Salad

Prep Time: 10–15 minutes ▪ Cook Time: 0 minutes ▪ Yield: 4 servings

Looking for a little intensity in your life? You can find it on your plate with this vibrant sweet and sour marriage of fruit and vegetables.

2 tablespoons fat-free plain Greek yogurt

Juice of 1 lime

2 tablespoons extra virgin olive oil

4 teaspoons champagne vinegar (or other light-tasting vinegar)

2 teaspoons agave nectar

2–3 cups arugula

½ jicama bulb, peeled and coarsely grated

½ Granny Smith apple (or other tart apple), coarsely grated or cut into thin slices

1 cup raspberries (or berries of personal preference)

In a small mixing bowl, whisk together yogurt, lime juice, oil, vinegar, and agave nectar. Separate out 1–2 tablespoons.

Toss together the arugula, jicama, and apple in a separate bowl. Toss well with the yogurt dressing (reserving the 1–2 separate tablespoons).

Plate onto 4 individual salad plates and top with berries. Drizzle with remaining dressing.

Black Bean, Corn, and Quinoa Salad

Prep Time: 15 minutes ▪ Cook Time: 0 minutes; Chill Time: several hours ▪ Yield: 4 servings

Fiber-rich, colorful, bursting with dynamic flavor, this is sure to become an all-time favorite recipe!

1 cup canned black beans

1 cup cooked quinoa

1 cup frozen sweet corn, thawed

½ cup finely chopped purple onion

½ cup chopped red bell pepper

1 medium-sized tomato, seeded and chopped

1 teaspoon salt

½ cup chopped cilantro (or parsley for a milder taste)

½ teaspoon dried basil (or 1 tablespoon finely chopped fresh basil)

2 tablespoons lime or lemon juice

1 tablespoon white balsamic vinegar (or apple cider vinegar)

In a large bowl combine all the ingredients and stir. Chill for at least half an hour and serve.

Celery Root Rémoulade

Prep Time: 20 minutes ▪ Cook Time: 0 minutes ▪ Yield: 4 servings

Creamy dressing and celery combine as a side dish solution for nearly any main dish.

1 pound celery root (celeriac)

1 ½ teaspoons salt

1 ½ teaspoons fresh lemon juice

3 tablespoons boiling water

¼ cup Dijon mustard

⅓–½ cup extra virgin olive oil

3 tablespoons white wine vinegar

Salt and freshly ground white pepper to taste

2–3 tablespoons minced fresh parsley

Peel the celery root with a vegetable peeler and cut into 1-inch chunks. Using a food processor, shred the celery root chunks into julienne slices. Immediately toss the shredded root in a large bowl with salt and lemon juice to prevent discoloration and to tenderize the root.

Meanwhile, pour the boiling water into a medium-sized bowl, add the mustard and whisk. Then add the oil, then the vinegar, and whisk again to make a thick, creamy sauce.

Rinse the celery root in cold water, drain, and dry. Fold it into the dressing, add salt and pepper, if needed, and sprinkle with parsley.

Fennel, Apple, and Arugula Salad

Prep Time: 15 minutes ▪ Cook Time: 0 minutes; Marinate Time: 30 minutes ▪ Yields: 4 servings

Fresh fennel's crispy crunch has the flavor of anise (licorice). Paired with crispy green apple and peppery arugula, this salad is anything but ordinary.

1 tablespoon white balsamic vinegar
Salt and pepper to taste
3 tablespoons olive oil
1 tablespoon fresh chopped parsley
2 small fennel bulbs
1 green apple
1 tablespoon freshly squeezed lemon juice
3 cups arugula
¼ cup grated Parmesan cheese
¼ cup roasted, unsalted almonds

In a small bowl, whisk the vinegar, salt, and pepper. Gradually whisk in the oil. Add the parsley and set aside.

Using a small, very sharp knife, remove the core at the base of the fennel bulbs and very thinly slice the bulbs. Core and thinly slice the apple and toss the apple with the lemon juice; set aside.

In a large bowl, toss together the fennel and apples and half of the dressing. Cover tightly and refrigerate for 30 minutes for the flavors to meld.

Add the arugula to the fennel mixture and toss gently with the remaining dressing. Arrange on 4 salad plates and sprinkle with the grated cheese and almonds.

Garlic Pita Chips

Prep Time: 15 minutes ▪ Cook Time: 10–12 minutes ▪ Yield: 6 servings

Tastier than any potato chip, and better for you, garlic pita chips are an ideal complement for soups and salads. Try them with the Hummus and Pesto Soup (page 166)!

1½ tablespoons olive oil
1 clove garlic, minced
1 teaspoon salt
½ teaspoon freshly ground black pepper
3 whole-wheat pita pockets, cut into 6 triangles each

Preheat the oven to 350°F. Place foil onto two large baking sheets.

In a small food processor or blender, combine the olive oil, garlic, salt, and pepper.

Open the pita pocket triangles to separate the tops from the bottoms and place the triangles on the baking sheets. Brush lightly with the olive oil seasoning mixture. Bake for 10–12 minutes or until golden brown. Let the pita chips cool on the baking sheets before handling.

Japanese Spinach Salad

Prep Time: 15 minutes ■ Cook Time: 2–3 minutes; Chill Time: 30 minutes ■ Yield: 2 servings

This is a simple and easy vitamin-rich side dish that goes well with main dishes such as Pan-Fried Wild Salmon and Mustard Sauce (page 189). Toasting the sesame seeds enhances the Asian flavor.

    Salt to taste
    1 pound fresh baby spinach (or 10 ounces frozen spinach)
    2 tablespoons plus 1 teaspoon toasted sesame seeds
    1 teaspoon sugar
    4 teaspoons low-sodium soy sauce
    1 tablespoon rice vinegar
    ½ teaspoon toasted sesame oil

Bring a large stockpot of salted water to a boil. Fill a medium bowl with ice cubes and water.

Add the fresh spinach to the pot and cook it for 20 seconds (if using frozen spinach, in a small saucepan, cook it in just a small amount of water until it falls apart). Remove the spinach (using either cooking method) and plunge into the ice water. After a few seconds, when the spinach has cooled, transfer it to a colander. Using your hands, squeeze as much of the water out of the spinach as you can. Spread the spinach out on a baking sheet lined with parchment paper and cover loosely with paper towels or a cloth towel. Chill in the refrigerator for half an hour.

In a dry small skillet over high heat, toast the sesame seeds, 2–3 minutes. Be sure to continuously shake the pan to prevent burning. Then, using a spice grinder or mortar and pestle, grind the sesame seeds with ½ teaspoon sugar.

In a medium bowl, combine the remaining ½ teaspoon sugar with the soy sauce, vinegar, and toasted sesame oil. Add the ground sesame seeds.

Add the chilled spinach and toss it with your hands to thoroughly combine with the spice mixture. Sprinkle with the remaining sesame seeds.

Mac and Cheese Cauliflower

Prep Time: 10–20 minutes ▪ Cook Time: 40 minutes ▪ Yield: 8 servings

This high-fiber, healthy twist on traditional mac and cheese gets the Overnight Diet seal of approval. Freeze leftovers in an airtight container and eat within 6–8 weeks.

1 large head cauliflower, broken into florets

2 tablespoons non-trans-fat buttery spread (I like Earth Balance)

3 tablespoons unbleached white flour

2 cups fat-free milk

2 cloves garlic, minced

1½ cups grated extra-sharp low-fat cheddar cheese

½ cup Parmesan cheese

½ cup nutritional yeast (*not* baker's or brewer's yeast) (I like Red Star or Bragg)

¼ teaspoon cayenne pepper

½ teaspoon paprika

1 egg

Nonstick cooking spray

½ cups prepared bread crumbs

Preheat the oven to 350°F. In a large stockpot, boil the cauliflower florets in salted water until tender, 5–7 minutes. Drain well and reserve 1 cup of the cooking liquid.

Using the same pot over medium heat, melt the buttery spread, whisk in the flour, and stir constantly for 1 minute. Whisk in the milk, garlic, and reserved cooking liquid, and cook 7–10 minutes or until the sauce is thickened, whisking constantly to prevent scorching. Remove from the heat, and stir in the cheese, nutritional yeast, cayenne pepper, paprika, and egg until the cheese is melted. Fold in the cauliflower.

Pour the mixture into a 13-by-9-inch baking dish coated evenly with nonstick cooking spray. Top with bread crumbs. Bake 30 minutes or until the casserole is hot and bubbly.

Rice Pilaf

Prep Time: 10 minutes ▪ Cook Time: 50 minutes ▪ Yield: 4 servings

Fragrant rice, lemony ginger, garlic, and Indian spices...who could ask for more?

    2 tablespoons extra virgin olive oil
    1 teaspoon mustard seeds
    1 medium yellow onion, chopped
    1 large carrot, coarsely grated
    1 tablespoon minced ginger
    4 garlic cloves, minced
    2 dried bay leaves
    ½ teaspoon turmeric
    1 teaspoon garam masala
    1 teaspoon salt
    2 cups brown basmati rice, rinsed
    ¼ cup golden raisins
    ¼ cup whole cashews or chopped almonds
    4 cups vegetable broth (I like low-sodium Frontier)
    1 cup chopped fresh cilantro

In a medium saucepan over medium-high heat, heat the oil, and when hot, add the mustard seeds. When they begin to pop, stir in the onion and carrot. Cook for a few minutes, until the onion begins to soften, and then stir in the ginger, garlic, bay leaves, turmeric, garam masala, and salt. Stir well, then add the rice, raisins, nuts, and broth. Stir well again, cover, bring to a boil, and simmer on low until cooked completely, 30–40 minutes.

When done, stir in the cilantro.

Roasted Garlic Cauliflower Mash

Prep Time: 20 minutes ▪ Cook Time: 45 minutes ▪ Yield: 4 servings

Roasted garlic is creamy, and cauliflower is a healthy replacement for the potato in mashed potatoes.

    1 bulb or head of garlic
    4 teaspoons extra virgin olive oil, divided in half

1 large head cauliflower, broken into small florets
⅓ cup low-fat buttermilk
2 tablespoons grated Parmesan cheese
1 teaspoon non-trans-fat buttery spread (I like Earth Balance)
1 tablespoon low-sodium vegetable broth powder
Salt and freshly ground black pepper to taste
Snipped fresh chives for garnish

Preheat the oven to 400°F. Peel away the outer papery layers of the garlic bulb skin. Leave the skin of each clove intact. Using a sharp knife, cut about ¼ inch off the top of the cloves so you can see the garlic inside the skin.

Place the bulb in a very small baking pan. Drizzle 2 teaspoons of the olive oil over the garlic head and use your fingers to coat the garlic cloves with oil. Cover the pan with aluminum foil.

Bake for 30 minutes or until the cloves are soft. The cloves will be very hot—let them cool before handling.

Use a small knife to cut into the cloves and squeeze the soft garlic out with your fingers.

Cook the cauliflower in a large saucepan with about an inch of water in the pan over medium-high heat until tender, 12–15 minutes. Drain well in a colander.

If using a food processor, combine the cauliflower with 2 teaspoons olive oil and the remaining ingredients except the chives in the bowl of the processor. If using an immersion blender, use a large bowl. Puree all the ingredients until thick and creamy.

Drizzle the remaining 2 teaspoons olive oil on top and garnish with chives.

Vanilla Poached Pears

Prep Time: 10 minutes ▪ Cook Time: 15–30 minutes ▪ Yield: 4 servings

Pears are in season during the late summer, fall, and early winter so you can enjoy this delicacy in all kinds of weather.

4 Bartlett or Bosc pears
Zest of 1 lemon
1–2 tablespoons freshly squeezed lemon juice (about ½ lemon)

2 tablespoons maple syrup
1 tablespoon sugar
1 teaspoon non-trans-fat buttery spread (I like Earth Balance)
1 teaspoon vanilla extract
1 cinnamon stick (optional)

Peel the pears, and using an apple corer, core them from the bottom and leave the stems on. Place the pears in a pot large enough to keep them upright, with lemon zest, lemon juice, and maple syrup, and cover with water (in winter, cinnamon brings a warming effect to desserts). Bring to a simmer and cook over low heat until tender when pierced with a knife, anywhere from 15 to 30 minutes. Remove from the heat and allow the pears to completely cool in the poaching liquid. Remove the pears to serving plates, and bring the poaching liquid to a fast boil. Stir in the sugar, buttery spread, and vanilla, and cook over low heat until the volume of the sauce has reduced to the desired consistency. Drizzle the sauce over and around pears. Serve warm.

DIPS, DRESSINGS, SPREADS, AND SAUCES

Avocado-Corn Salsa

Prep Time: 10 minutes ▪ **Cook Time: 0 minutes** ▪ **Yield: 2 servings**

This spicy salsa pairs well with baby carrots, zucchini, summer squash, and cucumber slices.

½ avocado, diced
½ cup frozen corn kernels, thawed
1 plum tomato, seeded and chopped
2 teaspoons fresh cilantro, chopped
Freshly squeezed lime juice to taste
Salt to taste

Combine the avocado, corn, tomato, and cilantro in a small bowl. Add the lime juice and salt to taste.

Basil Lime Sauce

Prep Time: 5 minutes ▪ Cook Time: 10 minutes ▪ Yield: 4 servings

Basil and lime together create a lively taste sensation that promises to brighten simple rice or pasta plates.

- 2 cups dry white wine
- 1–2 cloves garlic, minced
- 1 tablespoon finely minced shallot
- 2 teaspoons sugar
- 2 tablespoons freshly squeezed lime juice
- 1 cup chopped fresh basil
- 1 tablespoon non-trans-fat buttery spread
  (I like Earth Balance)

Place a medium skillet over medium-high heat and bring the wine, garlic, shallot, sugar, and lime juice to a boil, then immediately reduce the heat. Simmer until the sauce reduces by one-half in volume, 8–10 minutes. Turn off the heat and add the buttery spread; stir until melted. Let cool about 10 minutes and stir in the basil leaves.

Bean and Herb Dip

Prep Time: 5–7 minutes ▪ Cook Time: 0 minutes ▪ Yield: 8 servings

This is a hearty dip for vegetables or rice crackers, or a protein spread on a whole-wheat English muffin.

- 3 cloves garlic, minced
- 2 16-ounce cans cannellini beans, rinsed and drained
- 3 tablespoons lime or lemon juice
- 2 tablespoons olive oil
- 2 tablespoons chopped fresh basil
- 2 tablespoons chopped fresh parsley
- 1 tablespoon chopped fresh thyme or ½ teaspoon dried
- Salt and freshly ground black pepper to taste

In a food processor, puree all the ingredients until smooth and creamy.

Black Bean Hummus Spread

Prep Time: 5 minutes ▪ Cook Time: 0 minutes ▪ Yield: 8 servings

Legumes are a lip-smacking savory treat especially when blended with a little bit of olive oil and tahini. Spread on a whole-wheat tortilla and add sprouts, tomatoes, lettuce, onions, and any other vegetable of choice. Sure to be a hit!

    1 15-ounce can chickpeas, rinsed and drained
    1 15-ounce can black beans, rinsed and drained
    2 cloves garlic, minced
    1 tablespoon olive oil
    1 tablespoon tahini paste
    2 tablespoons lemon juice (more or less to taste)
    2 teaspoons cumin

In a food processor, pulse all ingredients for 2–3 minutes, until very smooth. Add water if needed to thin to desired consistency.

Buttermilk Dressing

Prep Time: 5 minutes ▪ Cook Time: 0 minutes ▪ Yield: 6–8 servings

Enjoy this modern take on old-fashioned buttermilk dressing, ideal for salads and dipping.

    ¾ cup fat-free mayonnaise
    ¾ cup low-fat buttermilk
    ½ teaspoon dried basil leaves
    Zest of 1 lemon
    1 teaspoon freshly squeezed lemon juice
    Salt and freshly ground black pepper to taste

In a small bowl, whisk together all the ingredients until smooth.

Cajun Hot Crab Dip

Prep Time: 15 minutes ▪ Cook Time: 30–35 minutes ▪ Yield: 12 ¼-cup servings

Everybody likes crab dip, especially when it's crunchy on top. Serve with fresh asparagus spears and green beans for a different type of vegetable-and-dip experience.

    Nonstick cooking spray
    2 tablespoons minced shallots

1 clove garlic, minced

1 pound lump crabmeat, divided

¼ cup water

1 tablespoon hot pepper sauce of choice

2 teaspoons salt-free Cajun seasoning

½ cup fat-free mayonnaise

⅓ cup fat-free cream cheese

¼ cup finely diced red bell pepper

2 tablespoons freshly squeezed lemon juice

Salt and freshly ground black pepper to taste

3 tablespoons panko bread crumbs

3 tablespoons finely sliced fresh chives or scallions

Preheat the oven to 450°F. Spray a small saucepan with nonstick cooking spray. Heat over medium heat. Add the shallots and garlic to the pan and cook for 2 minutes, stirring often to prevent scorching.

In a food processor, combine 1 cup crab meat, the shallot mixture, water, pepper sauce, and Cajun seasoning and process until smooth. Spoon the mixture into a large bowl, and stir in the remaining crab, the mayonnaise, cream cheese, bell pepper, lemon juice, salt, and pepper.

Lightly coat a 1-quart glass casserole dish with nonstick cooking spray and spoon the mixture into the dish. Combine the bread crumbs and chives in a small bowl and sprinkle over the crab mixture. Spray the bread crumb mixture with a little bit of cooking spray. Bake until lightly browned and bubbling, about 30 minutes. Let set for 5 minutes before serving.

Chili Lime Dressing

Prep Time: 5 minutes ▪ Cook Time: 0 minutes ▪ Yield: 6–8 servings

This dressing infuses salads with Asian-inspired flavor.

3 tablespoons low-sodium soy sauce

¼ cup freshly squeezed lime juice

2 tablespoons packed dark brown sugar

2 teaspoons Thai chili sauce

Whisk together all the ingredients in a small bowl.

Creamy Spinach Dip

Prep Time: 15 minutes ▪ Cook Time: 0 minutes ▪ Yield: 5 servings

Reinvent this all-time favorite spinach dip by using fat-free dairy.

1 small shallot, peeled
1 5-ounce can water chestnuts, rinsed and drained
½ cup fat-free cream cheese, softened
½ cup fat-free cottage cheese
¼ cup fat-free plain Greek yogurt
1 tablespoon lemon juice
Zest of ½ lemon
½ teaspoon salt
Freshly ground pepper to taste
Pinch of nutmeg
1 6-ounce package baby spinach
2 tablespoons chopped fresh chives

In a small food processor, pulse the shallot and water chestnuts until coarsely chopped. Add the cream cheese, cottage cheese, yogurt, lemon juice, lemon zest, salt, pepper, and nutmeg and pulse until just combined. Add the spinach and chives and pulse until creamy and smooth.

Honey Garlic Balsamic Vinaigrette

Prep Time: 5 minutes ▪ Cook Time: 0 minutes ▪ Yield: 6–8 servings

Sweet and slightly tangy, this robust dressing works with any salad.

6 tablespoons extra virgin olive oil
3 tablespoons aged balsamic vinegar
1 clove garlic, minced
½ teaspoon honey
2 tablespoons water

Pulse all the ingredients in a small food processor.

Lemon Caper Vinaigrette

Prep Time: 10 minutes ▪ Cook Time: 0 minutes ▪ Yield: 4 servings

Salty capers and astringent lemon make perfect companions in a sea of heart-healthy olive and flaxseed oils.

½ cup extra-virgin olive oil
¼ cup flaxseed oil
¼ cup white balsamic or champagne vinegar
4 teaspoons lemon juice
¼ cup capers, drained
Freshly ground pepper to taste

Combine all the ingredients thoroughly in a blender or salad dressing shaker to emulsify the oil and vinegar.

Low-Fat Edamame Dip

Prep Time: 5 minutes ▪ Cook Time: 5 minutes ▪ Yield: 8 servings

Edamame are a plant-based protein source that provide the base for this flavorful hummus-like dip for fresh, crispy vegetables.

1½ cups shelled and frozen edamame
1 tablespoon extra virgin olive oil
½ teaspoon salt
½ teaspoon ground cumin
2 garlic cloves, peeled
½ cup parsley leaves
3 tablespoons tahini
3 tablespoons water
3 tablespoons fresh lemon juice

Prepare the edamame according to package instructions but do not add any salt.

Place the olive oil, salt, cumin, and garlic in a food processor. Pulse a few times until coarsely chopped. Add the edamame, parsley, tahini, water, and lemon juice; process 1 minute or until smooth.

Orange and Avocado Salsa

Prep Time: 15 minutes ▪ Cook Time: 0 minutes ▪ Yield: 4 servings

Spoon this vibrant salsa over grilled chicken or wild salmon. Bursting with bright citrus flavor, creamy avocado, and the colorful taste of cilantro, it makes it seem like summer, no matter what time of year it is.

4 large oranges
2 large pink grapefruits
1 tablespoon minced jalapeño pepper

¼ cup finely minced red onion
2 tablespoons chopped fresh cilantro
2 teaspoons freshly squeezed lime juice
Salt to taste
1 diced peeled avocado

Peel the fruit, cut off the pith, and divide into sections. Cut the sections into small pieces.

Seed the jalapeño pepper and mince.

In a medium bowl, combine the fruit pieces, onion, cilantro, jalapeño, lime juice, salt, and avocado.

Salmon Spread

Prep Time: 10 minutes ▪ Cook Time: 0 minutes ▪ Yield: 12 ¼-cup servings

Use canned or leftover crumbled wild salmon for this tantalizing spread. Use rice crackers or fresh veggies for dipping.

1 14.75-ounce can pink salmon (without bones and skin)
1 3-ounce package fat-free cream cheese, softened
4 ounces plain fat-free Greek yogurt
1–2 teaspoons horseradish to taste
1 teaspoon lemon juice
Dash of seasoning mix (I like Spike)
2 teaspoons onion, grated or finely minced

In a medium-sized bowl, mix all the ingredients together, and press into a 16-ounce ramekin.

Savory Yogurt Dip

Prep Time: 5 minutes ▪ Cook Time: 0 minutes ▪ Yield: 1 serving

This peppery dip will spice up any crudité tray.

¼ cup fat-free Greek yogurt
Salt and freshly ground black pepper to taste
½ teaspoon lemon juice
¼ teaspoon lemon zest
1 tablespoon each of fresh thyme, dill, basil, and cilantro, chopped (or a few pinches each of dried)

In a small food processor, combine all the ingredients and pulse until smooth.

Sesame Miso Dressing

Prep Time: 5 minutes ▪ Cook Time: 0 minutes ▪ Yield: 6–8 servings

Try sesame miso dressing on your favorite salad when you're in the mood for an Asian-inspired dish.

⅓ cup rice wine vinegar

¼ cup white miso paste

2 tablespoons freshly squeezed lemon juice

2 teaspoons grated ginger

1 tablespoon organic sugar

2 tablespoons toasted sesame seeds + seeds to garnish

1 teaspoon toasted sesame oil

3 tablespoons mirin or cooking sake

Whisk together all the ingredients in a small bowl.

Spicy Blue Cheese Dip

Prep Time: 5 minutes ▪ Cook Time: 0 minutes ▪ Yield: 2 servings

There's a fusion of spice, creaminess, and crunch all in one bite. Serve with mounds of crunchy vegetables.

⅔ cup fat-free sour cream

⅔ cup crumbled low-fat blue cheese

1 tablespoon white wine vinegar

¼ teaspoon cayenne pepper (use just a pinch for less heat)

Whisk together all the ingredients in a small bowl.

Sweet and Spicy Sesame Dressing

Prep Time: 5 minutes ▪ Cook Time: 0 minutes ▪ Yield: 6–8 servings

Why decide between sweet and spicy? You can have both with this dressing.

2 tablespoons toasted sesame oil

1 tablespoon rice vinegar

1 tablespoon balsamic vinegar

1 teaspoon Sriracha or other chili-garlic sauce

1 teaspoon agave nectar

Whisk together all the ingredients in a small bowl.

Thai Peanut Dressing

Prep Time: 5 minutes ▪ Cook Time: 0 minutes ▪ Yield: 6–8 servings

If you're a fan of Thai food, you'll love this easy recipe for peanut dressing, a Thai staple.

1 cup low-sodium, fat-free chicken broth

2 tablespoons smooth natural peanut butter, no sugar added

1 tablespoon low-sodium soy sauce

1 teaspoon lime zest

2 tablespoons freshly squeezed lime juice

2 teaspoons toasted sesame oil

Whisk together all the ingredients in a small bowl.

Toasted Cumin Yogurt Dip

Prep Time: 10–15 minutes ▪ Cook Time: 1 minute; Chill Time: 1 hour–2 days ▪ Yield: 1 cup (2 servings)

Toast the cumin seeds in a dry skillet to enhance the flavor of this dip, and serve with vegetables, such as broccoli and cauliflower and carrots, for a zingy snack.

1 teaspoon cumin seeds

½ cup fat-free plain Greek yogurt

½ cup fat-free sour cream

1 small clove garlic, minced

¼ teaspoon salt

⅛ teaspoon cayenne pepper

In a small frying pan over high heat, toast the cumin seeds, shaking the pan constantly until fragrant, about 1 minute. Transfer the toasted seeds to a small bowl to cool.

In a medium bowl, combine the yogurt, sour cream, garlic, salt, and cayenne pepper.

Grind the toasted cumin seeds in a clean coffee grinder or with a mortar and pestle, or by mashing with the bottom of a small, heavy pan or mallet. Stir half the seeds into the dip, then add more to taste. Cover and chill to blend flavors for at least 1 hour and up to 2 days.

DESSERTS

Apple Cinnamon Brown Rice Pudding

Prep Time: 10 minutes ■ Cook Time: 1 hour 10 minutes ■ Yield: 4–6 servings

Although this sinless dessert takes a bit of pot watching and time, it's well worth the effort.

2 cups water
1 cup brown rice
Pinch of salt
4 cups fat-free milk
1 tablespoon agave nectar
3 tablespoons maple syrup
1 teaspoon vanilla extract
2 teaspoons ground cinnamon
Pinch each nutmeg and cloves
Generous ½ cup raisins
1 large apple, peeled, cored, seeded, and finely chopped

Combine the water, rice, and salt in a large Dutch oven or stockpot. Bring to a boil over medium-high heat, stir once, and cover with a tight-fitting lid. Reduce the heat to low and simmer for about 40 minutes or until most of the water is absorbed. Remove the rice from the heat, place in a bowl, and set aside.

To the same pot, add the milk, agave nectar, maple syrup, vanilla, cinnamon, nutmeg, and cloves. Bring to a very low boil over medium heat, stirring often so the milk doesn't burn, then reduce the heat to medium-low. Add in the cooked rice, raisins, and chopped apple. Cook over medium-low heat, stirring frequently. Reduce to low heat and simmer until the milk cooks down and the rice is creamy, about 30 minutes. Stir frequently to prevent scorching.

Portion out the pudding into 4–6 small ramekins. Serve warm or cold. If serving cold, cover with plastic wrap to prevent the pudding from forming a skin on top while refrigerating.

Apple Cranberry Crisp

Prep Time: 15 minutes ▪ Cook Time: 15 minutes ▪ Yield: 9 servings

The apple crisp gets a new slimmed-down look thanks to healthy, fiber-packed whole-wheat flour and oats.

   Nonstick cooking spray
   4 large sweet apples, peeled, cored, halved, and cut into thin slices
   ¼ cup dried naturally sweetened cranberries
   1 tablespoon water
   1 tablespoon and ¼ cup packed light brown sugar
   3 tablespoons whole-wheat flour
   2 tablespoons old-fashioned oats
   2 tablespoons non-trans-fat buttery spread (I like Earth Balance)

Preheat the oven to 450°F. Spray a 9-by-9-inch square baking pan with nonstick cooking spray.

In a large saucepan, combine the apples, cranberries, water, and 1 tablespoon brown sugar. Cook over medium-low heat until the apples begin to soften, 5–6 minutes. Stir occasionally to prevent sticking.

While the apples are cooking, combine the flour, oats, buttery spread, and remaining brown sugar in a small bowl. Use your fingers to mix until crumbly and set aside.

Place the hot apple mixture in the baking pan. Sprinkle the crumb mixture evenly on the top. Bake for 8–10 minutes, until lightly browned and hot throughout.

Cherries with Ricotta and Toasted Almonds

Prep Time: 2–4 minutes ▪ Cook Time: 5–6 minutes ▪ Yield: 2 servings

In just about 5 minutes, you can be enjoying a dessert that will remind you of cherry cheesecake.

   ¾–1 cup thawed frozen pitted sweet cherries

1 tablespoon water

2 tablespoons fat-free ricotta cheese

1–2 tablespoons toasted slivered almonds

In a small saucepan, heat the cherries with the water until they are warm, 5–6 minutes.

Transfer to a medium-sized ramekin or oven-safe bowl. Top the cherries with ricotta and almonds. (Optional: Slide the dessert under the broiler for just a few seconds—not too long or the almonds will burn.)

Figgy Cookie

Prep Time: 15 minutes ▪ Cook Time: 13 minutes ▪ Yield: 24 cookies (serving size: 2 cookies)

Remember Fig Newtons? These cookies are one up on goodness, flavor, and fiber. Enjoy without guilt.

½ cup non-trans-fat buttery spread (I like Earth Balance)

½ cup applesauce, unsweetened (I like Langers)

½ cup lightly packed brown sugar

½ cup sugar

4 tablespoons fat-free milk

1½ teaspoons vanilla extract

2¼ cups spelt or whole-wheat flour

1 teaspoon baking soda

Zest of ½ orange

1 teaspoon each of ground cinnamon and ginger

¾ cup old-fashioned rolled oats

¼ cup chocolate chips

½ cup sliced blanched almonds

⅓ cup finely diced dried figs

Preheat the oven to 350°F. Line a baking sheet with parchment paper. Combine the buttery spread, applesauce, sugars, milk, and vanilla extract in a bowl. Mix thoroughly. Add the flour, baking soda, orange zest, and spices. Stir until fully mixed, then stir in the oats, chocolate chips, nuts, and figs to make the dough.

Scoop spoonfuls of dough onto the baking sheet and flatten with the back of a spoon. Bake for 13 minutes or until golden.

Grandma's Low-Fat Chocolate Pudding

Prep Time: 10 minutes ▪ Cook Time: 15 minutes ▪ Yield: 4 servings

Diana's grandma made this recipe when Diana was little and it became the go-to after-dinner treat. The tradition continues.

½ cup sugar

3 tablespoons cornstarch

3 tablespoons dark chocolate cocoa, unsweetened (I like Now or Hershey's)

2½ cups fat-free milk

1½ teaspoons vanilla

In a small saucepan, over medium heat, combine the sugar, cornstarch, and cocoa. Gradually blend in the milk and continue cooking, stirring constantly, until the mixture thickens. Cook 3 minutes longer. Add the vanilla.

Pour into 4 ramekins or small dessert bowls and serve.

Granola Plum Mini-Muffin Pastries

Prep Time: 10 minutes ▪ Cook Time: 15–25 minutes ▪ Yield: 12 servings (2 muffins = 1 serving)

Flaxseeds, whole-wheat flour, and dried plums add a hint of fiber to these delicious dessert muffins.

¾ cup prunes

Boiling water

1 cup whole-wheat flour

½ cup unbleached white flour

1 cup fat-free or low-fat granola

¼ cup brown sugar

3 teaspoons baking powder

1 teaspoon cinnamon

½ teaspoon ground ginger

¼ cup ground flaxseeds

½ cup warm water

¼ cup molasses

2 teaspoons honey

2 tablespoons olive oil

2 tablespoons unsweetened applesauce (I like Langers)

1 cup fat-free milk
1 teaspoon vanilla extract
Nonstick cooking spray

Preheat the oven to 400°F. Chop the prunes into small bits and soak in a bowl with boiling water, filling just to cover. In a large bowl, combine the flours, granola, brown sugar, baking powder, cinnamon, and ginger; set aside.

In a small bowl, whisk together the flaxseeds and water. Add the molasses, honey, oil, applesauce, milk, and vanilla; set aside. Strain the prunes and stir into the flour mixture. Add the liquid mixture to the flour and stir just until moistened.

Spray 2 6-mini-muffin tins with nonstick cooking spray and spoon the batter into the wells until about two-thirds full. Bake for 10–15 minutes at 400°F, then lower the heat to 350°F and bake 5–10 minutes longer. The muffins are done when a toothpick inserted into the middle of a muffin comes out clean.

Grapes and Walnuts with Lemon Sour Cream Sauce

Prep Time: 20 minutes ▪ Cook Time: 0 minutes; Chill Time: 1–2 hours ▪ Yield: 4 servings

Here's the magic bullet for satisfying your sweet tooth with the fat-fighting duo of fruit and nuts.

½ cup fat-free sour cream
2 tablespoons powdered sugar
1 teaspoon lemon zest
1 teaspoon freshly squeezed lemon juice
⅛ teaspoon vanilla extract
1½ cups red seedless grapes
1½ cups green seedless grapes
3 tablespoons chopped walnuts

In a small bowl, whisk together the sour cream, powdered sugar, lemon zest, lemon juice, and vanilla. Cover and chill for 1–2 hours. Place the grapes in 4 wide-mouthed red wineglasses or ramekins. Add 2 tablespoons of the lemon topping to each dish and top with a sprinkle of chopped walnuts.

Grilled Fruit with Balsamic Syrup

Prep Time: 10–15 minutes ▪ Cook Time: 3–5 minutes ▪ Yield: 6 servings

Fruit is sweet—and it gets sweeter when it's HOT! Fire up the grill or broiler and get dessert going.

    1 small pineapple, peeled, cored, and cut into rings
    2 large mangoes, peeled and halved
    2 large peaches, pitted and halved
    1 tablespoon extra virgin olive oil
    2 tablespoons brown sugar
    ½ cup balsamic vinegar
    Nonstick cooking spray
    Mint or basil leaves, chopped for garnish

In a large bowl, combine the pineapple, mangoes, and peaches. Drizzle the olive oil over the fruit and stir or shake the bowl to coat each piece. Add the brown sugar and toss to coat evenly; set aside.

In a small saucepan, heat the balsamic vinegar on low. Simmer until the liquid is reduced in half, stirring occasionally to prevent burning. Remove from the heat; set aside.

Prepare the grill by spraying with nonstick cooking spray and heat to medium-high. Place the fruit on the grill racks. Grill until the fruit begins to brown, 3–5 minutes. Remove the fruit from the grill and arrange on individual serving plates. Drizzle with balsamic syrup and garnish with mint or basil.

Lemon Cheesecake Parfait

Prep Time: 5 minutes ▪ Cook Time: 0 ▪ Yield: 4 servings

This calcium-rich dessert is a sweet, flavorful, guiltless way to end dinner.

    4 full sheets graham crackers
    ½ cup part-skim or fat-free ricotta cheese
    1 ounce fat-free cream cheese
    2 tablespoons sugar
    1 6-ounce container fat-free lemon yogurt

Crush the graham crackers in a sealable plastic bag using a rolling pin or bottle.

In a blender, pulse the ricotta cheese, cream cheese, and sugar for 1 minute until well blended and smooth. Add the yogurt and pulse another 3–4 times. Avoid overmixing, or the cheese mixture will be too runny.

In 4 dessert cups or small stemless wineglasses, layer the ingredients, alternating graham cracker crumbs, cheese mixture, crumbs, and cheese mixture. Top with crumbs.

Lemon Custard with Fresh Blueberry Sauce

Prep Time: 15 minutes ▪ Cook Time: 1 hour 5 minutes; Chill Time: 4 hours ▪ Yield: 4 servings

Soft (or silken) tofu lends smoothness and silky texture to this custard. Blueberry sauce adds the sweet tang to balance the tartness of the lemon.

Nonstick cooking spray
½ cup silken tofu
1½ cups fat-free milk, divided into ½ cup and 1 cup
3 eggs
2 tablespoons firmly packed light brown sugar
2 tablespoons agave nectar
1 teaspoon lemon zest
½ teaspoon vanilla extract
½ teaspoon lemon extract
¼ cup all-fruit blueberry jam
2 tablespoons freshly squeezed lemon juice
¾ cup fresh blueberries

Preheat oven to 300°F. Spray four small ramekins with nonstick cooking spray.

In a blender or food processor, combine the tofu and ½ cup of the milk until smooth.

Meanwhile, in a small bowl, whisk the eggs thoroughly and add the brown sugar, agave nectar, lemon zest, and extracts. Whisk the egg mixture with the tofu mixture and 1 cup milk until well blended.

Pour the mixture into the ramekins and place them in a large baking pan filled halfway with hot water. Bake until the custards are set at the edge but are slightly loose at the center, about 50 minutes. Place the ramekins on a counter to finish setting, about 15 minutes. Cover with plastic wrap and chill at least 4 hours.

To make the blueberry sauce, whisk the jam and lemon juice in a small bowl until well blended. Stir in the blueberries gently to keep them intact. Top the custards with the blueberry sauce.

"On the Beam" Brownies

Prep Time: 10 minutes ▪ Cook Time: 30 minutes ▪ Yield: 12 servings

"On the beam" is a slang term for "brainy." Think of this as a smarter way to make brownies—they taste just as good and are good for you, too.

   Nonstick cooking spray
   12 ounces carrots
   7 ounces spinach
   1 box brownie mix (I like Arrowhead Mills, Duncan Hines, or Betty
      Crocker)
   ¼ cup extra virgin olive oil
   ¼ cup applesauce, unsweetened (I like Langers)
   2 eggs

Preheat the oven to 350°F. Spray an 8-by-8-inch baking dish with nonstick cooking spray. In a small food processor, puree 12 ounces of cooked carrots to yield ⅓ cup pureed; set aside. Cook the spinach to yield ⅓ cup pureed; set aside.

In a medium mixing bowl, combine the brownie mix, olive oil, applesauce, and eggs. Stir in the carrots and spinach and mix well. Pour the batter (it will be thick) into the dish and press into the corners. Bake for 30 minutes or until a toothpick inserted into the middle comes out clean.

Peachy Oat Crumble

Prep Time: 10 minutes ▪ Cook Time: 30 minutes ▪ Yield: 8 servings

Though it's designed for fresh and juicy August peaches, you can still enjoy this delectable crumble by using frozen peaches at other times of the year.

Nonstick cooking spray

8 ripe freestone peaches, peeled, pitted, and sliced (or 6 cups thawed frozen peaches)

Juice from 1 lemon

⅓ teaspoon ground cinnamon

¼ teaspoon ground nutmeg

½ cup whole-wheat flour

¼ cup packed dark brown sugar

2 tablespoons non-trans-fat buttery spread (I like Earth Balance)

¼ cup old-fashioned oats

Preheat the oven to 375°F. Lightly coat a 9-inch pie pan with nonstick cooking spray.

Arrange the peach slices in the pie plate. Sprinkle with lemon juice, cinnamon, and nutmeg.

In a small bowl, whisk together the flour and brown sugar. Using your fingers, crumble the buttery spread into the flour mixture. Add the oats and stir to mix evenly. Sprinkle the flour mixture evenly over the peaches.

Bake until the peaches are soft and bubbly and the topping is browned, about 30 minutes.

SPA BEVERAGES

Apple-licious Tonic

Prep Time: 5 minutes ▪ **Cook Time: 0 minutes** ▪ **Yield: 1 9-ounce serving**

A refreshing alternative to plain water.

1 ounce tart cherry juice (use small side of jigger to measure)

⅓ cup apple juice (store-bought)

⅓ cup orange juice (fresh-squeezed or store-bought)

⅓ cup pineapple juice (store-bought)

Ice, enough to fill shaker

Combine the cherry juice, apple juice, orange juice, and pineapple juice in a large shaker. Fill with ice and shake several minutes, until well chilled.

Basil Lime Spritzer

Prep Time: 10 minutes ▪ **Cook Time: < 1 minute** ▪ **Yield: 1 1-cup serving**

The idea of drinking basil may be new to you, but its peppery, licorice, and minty tastes create a unique combo of sweet and savory.

FOR THE SYRUP

1½ cups basil leaves
1 tablespoon + 2 teaspoons (or 6 packets total) Truvia
½ cup water
⅛ teaspoon baking soda

FOR THE SPRITZER

2 tablespoons freshly squeezed lime juice
Chilled sparkling water

In a small pot of boiling water, blanch the basil leaves for 8–10 seconds. Remove from the water with a slotted spoon and plunge right away into a bowl of ice water for 20 seconds to remove all heat. Remove from the water with the slotted spoon and drain well. In a blender, combine the basil, Truvia, water, and baking soda and puree for about 30 seconds. Strain the basil mixture through a fine mesh strainer (you can omit this step if you don't mind the basil pieces in your drink).

In a tall pitcher filled with ice, pour the basil syrup, lime juice, and sparkling water.

Cool Cucumber Cooler

Prep Time: 10 minutes ▪ **Cook Time: 3 minutes** ▪ **Yield: 8 servings**

Chilling, refreshing, light, and bright; the cucumber and lime notes in this spa drink are suitable for lazy summer afternoons.

½ cup water
3½ tablespoons (or 12 packets) Truvia
5 medium English cucumbers, peeled and coarsely chopped
4 cups cold water

1 1½-inch piece fresh ginger, peeled and chopped
½ cup freshly squeezed lime juice
4 cups ice

In a small saucepan, bring the water and Truvia to a boil, then let simmer until all the sugar substitute is dissolved, about 3 minutes, to make the simple syrup. (Use these same instructions to make the simple syrup in the Jalapeño Caipirinha, page 220.) Pour into a heat-resistant container to cool.

In a large blender or food processor, puree on high speed the cucumbers, water, and fresh ginger. Strain the cucumber mixture through cheesecloth into a pitcher and discard the solids. Stir in 4 tablespoons each of simple syrup and lime juice. Serve over ice.

Fuzzy Peach Sparkler

Prep Time: 2 minutes ▪ Chill Time: 0 ▪ Yield: 1 6-ounce serving

Enjoy this refreshing concoction any time of day—morning, noon, or night.

¼ cup peach nectar
6 ounces sparkling water (or diet tonic water for a sweeter taste)
Ice, enough to fill a large glass

In a large glass, combine the peach nectar, sparkling water, and ice. Stir until blended.

Iced White Tea

Prep Time: 5 minutes ▪ Steep Time: 3–5 minutes ▪ Yield: 4 1-cup servings

White tea's subtle flavor has been called soft, smooth, sweet, and sexy.

4 white tea bags (or about 12 teaspoons loose white tea)
5 cups water
1 tablespoon + 2 teaspoons (or 6 packets total) Truvia
4 fresh mint leaves + extra for garnishing

Steep the tea bags or loose tea in 4 cups boiling water for 3–5 minutes, then chill.

While chilling, bring a cup of water, the sugar substitute, and the mint leaves to a boil, remove from the heat, and let steep until cool.

Sweeten the tea with the mint syrup to taste and garnish with mint leaves.

Jalapeño Caipirinha

Prep Time: 5 minutes ▪ Cook Time: 3 minutes ▪ Yield: 1 12-ounce serving

Inspired by the national cocktail of Brazil, this "mocktail" offers a South American spiciness.

1 lime
½ fresh jalapeño
2 ounces simple syrup (see instructions in Cool Cucumber Cooler recipe, page 218)
Ice, enough to fill shaker
Sparkling water

Cut the lime in half, squeeze well, then cut the lime peel into quarters. Cut the jalapeño in half lengthwise and remove the seeds. In a shaker, combine the lime juice, jalapeño, and simple syrup. Fill with ice, and shake vigorously. Pour into a 12-ounce glass, and top off with sparkling water.

Pomegranate Nectar

Prep Time: 5 minutes ▪ Cook Time: 0 minutes ▪ Yield: 1 12-ounce serving

Pomegranate juice is full of healthy antioxidants, and even better, it tastes great.

¼ cup pomegranate juice
¾ cup mango nectar
4 ounces sparkling water

In a large glass, combine the pomegranate juice, mango nectar, and sparkling water. Stir until blended.

Pomegranate Splashers

Prep Time: 5 minutes ▪ Cook Time: 0 minutes ▪ Yield: 1 10-ounce serving

The splash of lime adds a twist to the pomegranate juice.

¼ cup pure pomegranate juice
1 cup sparkling water

1 teaspoon lime juice
Ice, enough to fill a large glass

In a large glass, combine the pomegranate juice, sparkling water, lime juice, and ice. Stir until blended.

Shirley Temple

Prep Time: 10 minutes ▪ Cook Time: 1 hour 5 minutes; Cooling Time: 30 minutes ▪ Yield: 6 servings

Add pomegranate syrup to just about any beverage to create your favorite "mocktail."

¼ cup pomegranate syrup (recipe below)
8 ounces diet ginger ale
Maraschino cherry

In a large glass, combine the syrup and ginger ale. Stir until blended. Garnish with the cherry.

POMEGRANATE SYRUP

4 cups pomegranate juice
3½ tablespoons (or 12 packets) Truvia
1 tablespoon freshly squeezed lemon juice

In a small saucepan over medium heat, bring the pomegranate juice, Truvia, and lemon juice to a boil. Cook, stirring frequently, until the sugar substitute has completely dissolved. Then, reduce the heat to medium-low and cook until the mixture has reduced to about 1½ cups, nearly the consistency of syrup. This will take about an hour. Remove from the heat and cool for 30 minutes.

Transfer to a glass jar and cool completely. Cover and store in the refrigerator for up to 3 months.

Sparkling Watermelon Sipper

Prep Time: 10 minutes ▪ Chill Time: 3 hours ▪ Yield: 8 1-cup servings

Summertime is best with refreshing watermelon—this time in a glass!

10 cups peeled watermelon chunks

3 cups cold water
⅓ cup freshly squeezed lime juice
1 tablespoon + 2 teaspoons (or 6 packets total) Truvia
Ice cubes, enough to fill a glass
8 lime wedges

Using a blender, purée ⅓ of the watermelon and water in three separate batches; pour each batch into a large pitcher to hold. Add the lime juice and Truvia to the watermelon mixture in each pitcher and stir until well blended. Refrigerate until very chilled, at least 3 hours. When ready to serve, pour over glasses filled with ice cubes. Garnish each glass with a lime wedge if desired.

Spiced Ginger Lemon Spritzer

Prep Time: 5 minutes ■ Cook Time: 1 hour ■ Yield: 6 12-ounce servings

Ginger has long been used as a tummy tonic for easy digestion and to quell queasiness. Enjoy this mocktail as an after-dinner tonic.

Fresh ginger, 4-inch piece
Zest of 2 lemons
3–4 cinnamon sticks
½ teaspoon cloves
¼ teaspoon nutmeg
⅔ cup + 3 tablespoons Truvia
1 cup water
2 liters sparkling water (or diet tonic water for a sweeter taste)
6 lemon slices

Peel then cut the fresh ginger into 1-inch pieces. In a small saucepan, bring to a quick boil the ginger, lemon zest, cinnamon sticks, cloves, nutmeg, Truvia, and water. Lower the heat and simmer for 30 minutes. Strain into a small pitcher and cool.

For each drink, add 2 ounces of the syrup to a serving glass and top with sparkling water. Garnish with a slice of lemon.

Virgin Mojito

Prep Time: 5 minutes ■ Chill Time: 0 ■ Yield: 1 12-ounce serving

This mocktail is so tasty, you could serve it at a party!

½ of 1 lime, cut into small pieces
6 large mint leaves
¾ teaspoon Truvia
Ice, enough to fill a 12-ounce glass
12 ounces sparkling soda

In a 12-ounce glass, muddle (mash to release the juice and flavors) the lime, mint, and sugar substitute. Nearly fill the glass with ice and top off with the sparkling soda. Stir lightly.

CHAPTER 9

Quickie Rev Up Moves and Routines

Are you ready to resculpt your body so you can have long, lean muscles and a slimmer, sexier shape? In this chapter, you will see just how easy it can be to maintain muscle mass so you can boost your metabolism and blast fat faster than ever. With the unique two-in-one Quickie Rev Up routine, all it takes is 21 minutes, just four times a week. A 3-minute Dynamic Warm Up primes your body from head to toe and then you alternate between 60-second Rev Up Blasts and 2 minutes of Strength Training Moves. How simple is that?

All you have to do is move through the routine quickly without taking any breaks. Be sure to start at the appropriate level to reduce the risk of injury and maximize results. The table below shows the basic structure of what your workout will look like each time you complete it.

Quickie Rev Up Structure

Dynamic Warm Up	3 minutes
Strength Training Move	2 minutes
Rev Up Blast	1 minute
Strength Training Move	2 minutes
Rev Up Blast	1 minute
Strength Training Move	2 minutes
Rev Up Blast	1 minute

Strength Training Move	2 minutes
Rev Up Blast	1 minute
Strength Training Move	2 minutes
Rev Up Blast	1 minute
Strength Training Move	2 minutes
Rev Up Blast	1 minute

Remember, you will have the option to adjust the difficulty of the moves based on your fitness level as determined by the assessment on pages 101–104.

- **Make It Easier:** If you answered mostly A's on the assessment, start with the "Make It Easier" versions of the Quickie Rev Up Foundation Moves for at least two weeks.
- **Basic Move:** If you answered mostly B's on the assessment, start with the "Basic Move" options of the five Quickie Rev Up Foundation Moves for at least two weeks.
- **Rev It Up:** If you answered mostly C's on the assessment, start with the "Rev It Up" versions of the five Quickie Rev Up Foundation Moves for at least two weeks.

Never feel pressured to advance to the next level before you're ready. This is not a race!

Check with your physician before starting any exercise program.

Quickie Rev Up Vocab Lesson

Athletic stance: You don't have to be a professional athlete to assume an athletic stance. But mastering this simple posture while working out can boost your performance and help reduce the risk of injury. Here's how you do it: Stand with your feet approximately hip-width apart and your knees slightly bent as you look straight ahead and keep your shoulders down, your chest out, and your back straight.

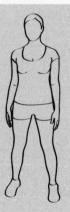

Split stance: Start in an athletic stance, then keeping your feet hip-width apart, step one foot about 18 to 24 inches forward. Make sure your front foot is flat on the floor while your back one is resting on the ball of the foot.

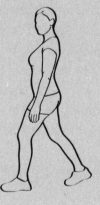

Dynamic Warm Up Moves

Do the following five Dynamic Warm Up moves in sequence for a total of 3 minutes.

Twisting High Knees

What It Works: Front Thighs, Midsection

1. Start in an athletic stance with your arms bent in front of you so your hands are level with your shoulders.

2. Raise your left knee in front of
   you as you twist your upper
   body toward it, reaching the
   elbow toward the knee.
3. Lower your left leg and return
   to the starting point.
4. Repeat on the right side, raising
   your right knee and twisting to
   the right. This completes one rep.
5. Keep alternating sides for
   30 seconds.

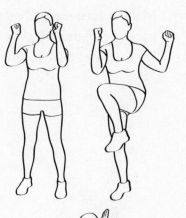

Make It Easier: Instead of touching your elbow to
your knee, touch your hands to your knee.

Butt Kicks

What It Works: Rear Thighs

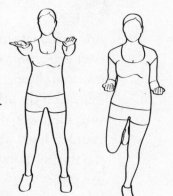

1. Start in an athletic stance but with
   your feet wider than hip-width
   apart and hold your arms straight
   out in front of you at shoulder height.
2. In one fluid motion, bend your
   arms and bring both of your elbows
   in to your sides and swing your
   right heel up behind you so it
   touches—or comes close to—your butt.
3. Bring your arms back out to shoulder height and your right
   foot back to the floor.
4. Repeat on the left side by pulling your arms in to your sides
   and bringing your left heel to your butt then back down to
   the floor.
5. Keep alternating from side to side for 30 seconds.

Make It Easier: Hold on to the back of a chair with two hands as you raise your feet.

Heel Touches

What It Works: Front Thighs, Midsection

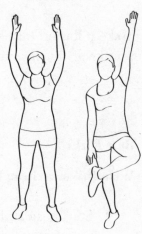

1. Start in an athletic stance with your arms raised over your head.
2. In one motion, lift your left foot in front of you and angle your left knee out to the side while you bring your right hand down to touch your left heel.
3. Bring your left foot back down to the floor and raise your arm back up over your head.
4. Repeat on the other side, raising your right foot and touching it with your left hand, then returning to the starting point. This completes one rep.
5. Keep alternating from side to side for 30 seconds.

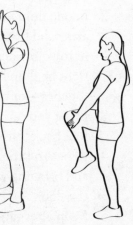

Make It Easier: Start with your arms out to your sides at shoulder height, elbows bent, and touch the inside of your knee instead of your ankle.

Lateral Leg Swings

**What It Works: Inner and Outer
Thighs, Midsection**

1. Start by balancing on your
left foot with your right foot
hovering just off the floor in
front of you and your arms
out to the sides for balance.
2. Swing your right leg to the left
as if you were using your foot
to push a door closed as you
swing your arms in the opposite direction.
Your arms will help you balance. If you
have trouble balancing, feel free to touch
a counter or the wall for support.
3. Without stopping, swing your leg
back to the right as high as you can
comfortably as your arms swing
to the left. This completes one rep.
4. Swing your right leg from side to side for
30 seconds, then switch sides and swing your left leg from
side to side for 30 seconds.

Make It Easier: Hold on to the back of a chair with one hand and
place the other on your hip.

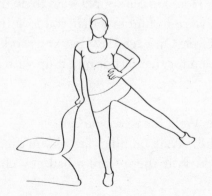

Frankenstein March

What It Works: Front Thighs, Rear Thighs

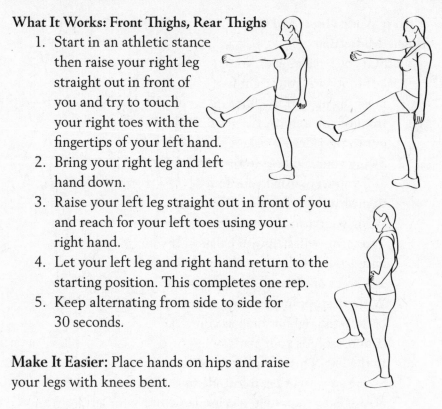

1. Start in an athletic stance then raise your right leg straight out in front of you and try to touch your right toes with the fingertips of your left hand.
2. Bring your right leg and left hand down.
3. Raise your left leg straight out in front of you and reach for your left toes using your right hand.
4. Let your left leg and right hand return to the starting position. This completes one rep.
5. Keep alternating from side to side for 30 seconds.

Make It Easier: Place hands on hips and raise your legs with knees bent.

Rev Up Blasts

These 60-second blasts will get your heart pumping and will fire up your metabolism. Here are ten simple ways to do the 60-second Rev Up Blasts. You're sure to find one that you love that is appropriate for your fitness level. On each day that you work out, choose one Rev Up Blast option for that day or mix it up with multiple options. It's up to you.

1. **Walk Fast:** Walk as fast as you can.
2. **Walk Uphill:** Walk uphill as fast as you can.
3. **Sprint:** Run as if there were a bad guy chasing you with a knife.

4. **Walk/Jog Up Stairs:** Walk briskly or jog up stairs. When this feels comfortable, try taking two stairs at a time.
5. **Jog in Place:** Bring your knees up high to your chest as you jog in place.
6. **Step Up and Down:** Step up on a stair or curb with one foot, then the other foot, then step down one foot at a time. Keep stepping up and down as quickly as possible.
7. **Repeaters:** Step up on a stair or curb with one foot, making sure that your standing leg is bent. Bring the knee of your other leg up to your chest then back down, lightly tapping your foot on the floor before raising your knee back up. Keep raising and lowering your knee for 30 seconds. Then switch sides, stepping off the step and bringing your other foot onto the step and raising the opposite knee, for the remaining 30 seconds.
8. **Jumping Jacks:** You know the drill. If you aren't ready for jumping jacks, start in an athletic stance and instead of jumping, simply rise up onto your toes as you swing your arms overhead.
9. **Quick Feet:** This is similar to a drill commonly used in football training. Starting from an athletic stance but with your feet wider than hip-width apart, lean your upper body slightly forward and run in place as quickly as you can.
10. **Toe Touch Jumps:** Start from an athletic stance but with your feet wider than hip-width apart and raise both arms up over your head. Crouch down and touch your toes, then jump as you rise back up and raise your arms back up over your head. Make sure your knees are slightly bent when you land and immediately go back into your crouch.

Workout Tip

Breathe Easy! Many people tend to hold their breath while working out, but this habit can cause light-headedness, may cause you to strain your back, and can make exercises seem even harder than they are. Remembering to breathe normally helps prevent injuries and eases you through challenging exercises.

Strength Training Moves

Regardless of your fitness level, it is best to master the five Quickie Rev Up Basic Foundation Moves before tackling the Quickie Rev Up Advanced Moves.

Quickie Rev Up Foundation Moves

Bridge

What It Works: Buttocks, Rear Thighs, and Muscles That Support the Lower Back
  Basic Move:

1. Lie on your back on the floor and bend your knees.
2. Tuck your pelvis under and lift your hips off the floor. Form a straight slope with your body from your shoulders to your knees.
3. Hold for 30 seconds, then relax for 10 seconds. Repeat two more times.

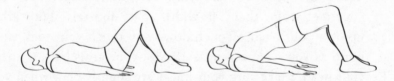

Make It Easier: Don't lift your hips off the floor. Just tuck your pelvis so you feel your back make contact with the floor.

Rev It Up: With your hips lifted, raise your right foot off the floor and straighten your right leg, keeping it parallel to your left leg. Hold for 15 seconds, then bring your right foot back down and straighten your left leg and hold for another 15 seconds. Bring your left foot back down and rest for 10 seconds before repeating the sequence.

Plank

What It Works: Midsection, Chest, Front Shoulders, Rear Arms
Basic Move:

1. Lie facedown with toes tucked under and forearms on the floor.
2. Pull your belly up and in and raise hips off the floor so your body forms a straight line from your shoulders to your hips— a plank. Your elbows should be bent at a 90-degree angle directly under your shoulders. Keep your back straight— don't let your butt pop up in the air or let your hips sag down toward the floor.
3. Squeeze your midsection in constantly and hold this position. Don't forget to breathe.
4. Hold for 30 seconds, then relax for 10 seconds. Repeat two more times.

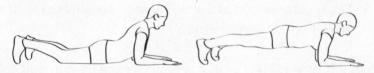

Make It Easier: Drop your knees to touch the floor while maintaining your alignment.

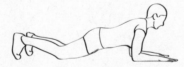

Rev It Up: Straighten your arms into a full push-up position while maintaining your alignment.

Quickie Rev Up Vocab Lesson

Core Versus Midsection What's the difference between your core and your midsection? Your midsection is what you typically think of as your abs—the muscles in your abdomen and on the sides of your waist. Your core also includes a group of muscles that support your back.

Squat

What It Works: Buttocks, Front Thighs, Rear Thighs, Core
Basic Move:

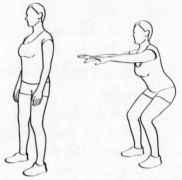

1. Start in an athletic stance and contract your midsection as you lower your butt as if you were going to sit in a chair. Don't let your hips sink lower than knees and don't let your knees jut farther forward than your toes. Reach forward with your arms for balance.
2. Contract your buttocks and thighs to press back up to standing.
3. Do as many as you can in 30 seconds, then relax for 10 seconds. Repeat two more times.

Make It Easier: Place a chair behind you and let your butt touch the chair momentarily before coming back to standing.

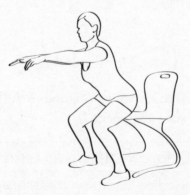

Rev It Up: As you come back to standing, raise your arms overhead or add a jump.

Lunge

What It Works: Calves, Rear Thighs, Front Thighs, Inner and Outer Thighs, Buttocks
   Basic Move:

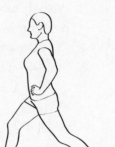

1. Start in a split stance with your right foot in front.
2. Lower your hips until your left knee is almost touching the floor. Make sure your right knee is in line with your right toes, but not in front of them.
3. Engage the muscles in your legs to come back up to standing.
4. Do as many reps as you can in 30 seconds, then switch sides and repeat for 30 seconds. Repeat one more time on each side.

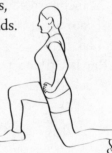

   Make It Easier: Don't lower your hips as much.
   Rev It Up: When you come back to standing, raise both arms overhead.

Push-Up

What It Works: Chest, Front Shoulders, Rear Arms, Midsection
   Basic Move:

1. Start in a push-up position with the palms of your hands on the floor slightly wider than your shoulders and your knees touching the floor. Pull your midsection in and keep your body in a straight line from your knees to your head as in a plank. Don't let your butt pop up in the air or sag down to the floor.
2. Bend your elbows as you lower yourself down toward the floor, keeping your body in that straight line.

3. Push back up to the start position, maintaining the same position with your body.

4. Do as many as you can in 30 seconds, then relax for 10 seconds. Repeat two more times.

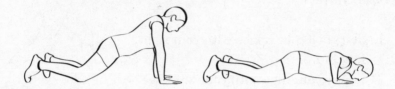

Make It Easier: Instead of lying facedown, stand facing a wall and place the palms of your hands on the wall at shoulder level but slightly wider than your shoulders. Move your feet back 12–24 inches so you are leaning at an angle. Push against the wall until your arms are fully extended then return to the starting position.

Rev It Up: Start with your knees lifted off the floor and your toes tucked under.

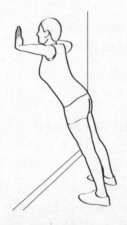

Workout Tip

Bend It To reduce the risk of injury, avoid locking out your knees and elbows while strength training. Maintain a slight bend to protect your joints.

Advanced Quickie Rev Up Moves

Wall Sit

What It Works: Front Thighs, Rear Thighs, Buttocks, Calves
Basic Move:

1. With your back flat against a wall, and your feet hip-width apart about 2 feet away from the wall, slide down until your hips are at a 90-degree angle and your knees are directly over your ankles. Adjust your feet if necessary so that your knees are aligned with your ankles.
2. Hold the position for 30 seconds, then relax for 10 seconds. Repeat two more times.

Make It Easier: Don't slide down the wall quite as far.

Rev It Up: Hold the position for 50 seconds, then relax for 10 seconds. Repeat one more time.

Side Plank

What It Works: Midsection, Shoulders, Rear Arms, Core
Basic Move:

1. Lie on your left side with your left forearm on the floor and your elbow directly below your left shoulder. Keep your legs straight with your right leg stacked directly on top of your left leg.

2. Pull in your midsection as you lift your hips and knees off the floor to create a straight line with your body. Keep your head in line with your spine and don't let your hips pop up in the air or sag toward the floor.

3. Hold for 30 seconds, then return to the start position and switch to the other side. Repeat one more time on each side.

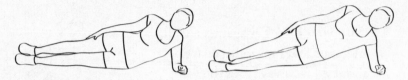

Make It Easier: Put your right knee on the floor in front of the left for stability.

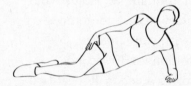

Rev It Up: With your hips lifted off the floor, raise your upper leg a few inches off your lower leg and raise the arm that isn't supporting you toward the ceiling to form a star.

Walking Lunge

What It Works: Calves, Front Thighs, Rear Thighs, Inner and Outer Thighs, Hips, Buttocks
Basic Move:

1. Start in an athletic stance.
2. Step forward with your left foot and lower your hips until your right knee is almost touching the floor. Make sure your left knee does not jut past your left toes.
3. In one fluid motion, engage the muscles in your legs and come back up to standing as you step forward with your right foot.

4. Lower your hips until your left knee is almost touching the floor. Make sure your right knee does not jut past your right toes.
5. Keep alternating sides as you walk and lunge.
6. Do as many reps as you can in 30 seconds, then relax for 10 seconds. Repeat two more times.

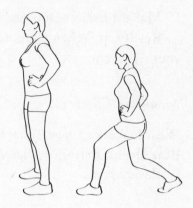

Make It Easier: Don't lower your hips as much.

Rev It Up: When you come back to standing, pull the knee of your back leg up to your chest and raise your opposite arm over your head.

Lunge and Twist

What It Works: Calves, Front Thighs, Rear Thighs, Inner and Outer Thighs, Buttocks, Midsection, Core
Basic Move:

1. Start in a split stance with your left foot forward and bend your arms so your hands are in line with your shoulders.
2. Lower your hips until your right knee comes close to the floor. At the same time, twist your upper body to the left.
3. Return to the start position.
4. Do as many reps as you can in 30 seconds, then switch sides and repeat for 30 seconds. Repeat one more time on each side.

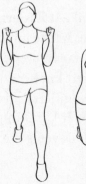

Make It Easier: Don't go as low when you lunge.

Rev It Up: When you rotate your upper body to the left, extend your right arm.

Mountain Climbers

What It Works: Chest, Front Shoulders, Rear Arms, Front Thighs, Rear Thighs, Buttocks, Midsection
Basic Move:

1. Start in a push-up position with your arms extended, your hands directly under your shoulders, and your toes tucked under. Keep your body in a straight line, not allowing your butt to pop up in the air or sag down to the floor.
2. Bring your right knee in toward your chest and let the ball of your right foot touch the floor.
3. Return to the start position then bring your left knee in toward your chest and let the ball of your left foot touch the floor.
4. Alternate from side to side for 30 seconds, then relax for 10 seconds. Repeat two more times.

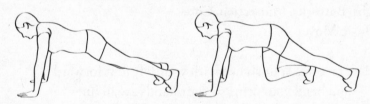

Make It Easier: Start in an athletic stance. At the same time, raise your right arm straight over your head and lift your left knee. Return to start then raise your left arm and right knee.

Rev It Up: Jump and switch feet in the air as you go from side to side.

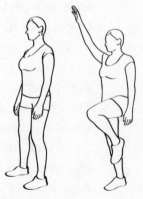

Take Your Quickie Rev Up to the Gym

If you prefer to work out at a gym, then by all means, take your Quickie Rev Up to the nearest one. For added variety, you can work the same muscles using equipment you will find at most gyms. As with this program's body weight moves, you can adapt the exercises you do on machines to your fitness level. To make moves easier, use lighter weight or do fewer repetitions. To rev it up, use heavier weights or perform more repetitions.

Strength Training Recommendations for Resistance Machines

Exercise Selection	Perform 8–10 resistance machine exercises that cumulatively engage all the major muscle groups.
Exercise Resistance	Use a resistance that enables you to complete at least 8 repetitions but not more than 12 repetitions.
Exercise Progression	Increase the exercise resistance by approximately 5% whenever you complete 12 or more repetitions.
Exercise Sets	Perform one perfect set of each exercise.
Exercise Speed	Use a controlled movement speed of approximately 6 seconds per repetition, with 3 seconds for each lifting action and 3 seconds for each lowering action.
Exercise Range	Use a complete movement range for each repetition, but never push yourself into painful positions.
Exercise Breathing	Exhale during lifting actions and inhale during lowering actions; never hold your breath.

Here is a quick look at the gym equipment that is best to use and the area of the body that each machine works. If you aren't familiar with these machines, ask a personal trainer or a gym employee for assistance in using them.

- Leg extension machine (front thighs)
- Leg curl machine (rear thighs)
- Leg press machine (front thighs, rear thighs, buttocks)
- Chest press machine (chest, front shoulders, rear arms)
- Pull down machine (upper back, front arms, forearms)
- Shoulder press machine (shoulders, rear arms)
- Mid-row machine (upper back, front arms, forearms)
- Abdominal machine (midsection)
- Low back machine (core)
- Rotary torso machine (midsection)

Keep It Revved Up

After just two weeks of doing the Quickie Rev Up, you will start to feel stronger, more energized, and more toned. You will be losing pounds without losing the lean muscle mass that gives your body definition. When you see results so quickly, it keeps you motivated, which makes it so much easier to stick with the routine. And when you regularly devote 21 minutes four times a week to the Quickie Rev Up, it keeps fat burning and weight loss revved up, too.

2-WEEK QUICKIE REV UP PLAN—BASIC MOVES

WEEK 1

Day 1 1-Day Power Up	Day 2 6-Day Fuel Up	Day 3	Day 4	Day 5	Day 6	Day 7
	Dynamic Warm Up		Dynamic Warm Up		Dynamic Warm Up	Dynamic Warm Up
	Basic Bridge		Basic Push-Up		Basic Lunge	Basic Plank
	Walk Fast		Jog in Place		Walk Fast	Jog in Place
	Basic Plank		Basic Squat		Basic Bridge	Basic Push-Up
	Walk Fast		Jog in Place		Walk Fast	Jog in Place
R&R	Basic Squat	R&R	Basic Plank	R&R	Basic Squat	Basic Plank
	Walk Fast		Jog in Place		Walk Fast	Jog in Place
	Basic Push-Up		Basic Lunge		Basic Lunge	Basic Push-Up
	Walk Fast		Jog in Place		Walk Fast	Jog in Place
	Basic Lunge		Basic Push-Up		Basic Bridge	Basic Plank
	Walk Fast		Jog in Place		Walk Fast	Jog in Place
	Basic Plank		Basic Squat		Basic Squat	Basic Push-Up
	Walk Fast		Jog in Place		Walk Fast	Jog in Place

continued

2-WEEK QUICKIE REV UP PLAN—BASIC MOVES (continued)

WEEK 2

Day 1 1-Day Power Up	Day 2 6-Day Fuel Up	Day 3	Day 4	Day 5	Day 6	Day 7
	Dynamic Warm Up		Dynamic Warm Up		Dynamic Warm Up	Dynamic Warm Up
	Basic Squat		Basic Push-Up		Basic Lunge	Basic Push-Up
	Step Up and Down		Repeaters		Step Up and Down	Repeaters
	Basic Lunge		Basic Bridge		Basic Squat	Basic Plank
	Step Up and Down		Repeaters		Step Up and Down	Repeaters
R&R	Basic Plank	R&R	Basic Plank	R&R	Basic Bridge	Basic Plank
	Step Up and Down		Repeaters		Step Up and Down	Repeaters
	Basic Squat		Basic Lunge		Basic Lunge	Basic Push-Up
	Step Up and Down		Repeaters		Step Up and Down	Repeaters
	Basic Lunge		Basic Push-Up		Basic Squat	Basic Plank
	Step Up and Down		Repeaters		Step Up and Down	Repeaters
	Basic Plank		Basic Squat		Basic Bridge	Basic Plank
	Step Up and Down		Repeaters		Step Up and Down	Repeaters

2-WEEK QUICKIE REV UP PLAN—ADVANCED MOVES

WEEK 1

Day 1 1-Day Power Up	Day 2 6-Day Fuel Up	Day 3	Day 4	Day 5	Day 6	Day 7
	Dynamic Warm Up		Dynamic Warm Up		Dynamic Warm Up	Dynamic Warm Up
	Walking Lunges		Mountain Climbers		Basic Squat	Mountain Climbers
	Quick Feet		Jumping Jacks		Sprint	Walk Uphill
	Side Plank		Basic Lunge		Lunge and Twist	Side Plank
	Quick Feet		Jumping Jacks		Sprint	Walk Uphill
R&R	Basic Squat	R&R	Side Plank	R&R	Wall Sit	Basic Push-Up
	Quick Feet		Jumping Jacks		Sprint	Walk Uphill
	Mountain Climbers		Lunge and Twist		Basic Lunge	Basic Plank
	Quick Feet		Jumping Jacks		Sprint	Walk Uphill
	Wall Sit		Basic Plank		Basic Squat	Side Plank
	Quick Feet		Jumping Jacks		Sprint	Walk Uphill
	Basic Push-Up		Basic Squat		Walking Lunges	Basic Push-Up
	Quick Feet		Jumping Jacks		Sprint	Walk Uphill

continued

2-WEEK QUICKIE REV UP PLAN—ADVANCED MOVES (continued)

WEEK 2

Day 1 1-Day Power Up	Day 2 6-Day Fuel Up	Day 3	Day 4	Day 5	Day 6	Day 7
R&R	Dynamic Warm Up	R&R	Dynamic Warm Up	R&R	Dynamic Warm Up	Dynamic Warm Up
	Mountain Climbers		Walking Lunges		Basic Squat	Mountain Climbers
	Jog Up Stairs		Toe Touch Jumps		Repeaters	Sprint
	Walking Lunges		Basic Plank		Lunge and Twist	Side Plank
	Quick Feet		Jog in Place		Jumping Jacks	Quick Feet
	Basic Push-Up		Basic Squat		Wall Sit	Basic Push-Up
	Jog Up Stairs		Toe Touch Jumps		Step Up and Down	Jog Up Stairs
	Side Plank		Side Plank		Walking Lunges	Basic Plank
	Quick Feet		Jog in Place		Repeaters	Sprint
	Lunge and Twist		Wall Sit		Basic Squat	Mountain Climbers
	Jog Up Stairs		Toe Touch Jumps		Jumping Jacks	Quick Feet
	Mountain Climbers		Basic Push-Up		Basic Lunge	Basic Plank
	Quick Feet		Jog in Place		Step Up and Down	Jog Up Stairs

PART IV

THE

OVERNIGHT

DIET FOR LIFE!

CHAPTER 10

The Overnight Diet Eating Out Guide

Life is full of happy, exciting occasions. And the vast majority of them center around—you guessed it—food. Going out to dinner with friends, sharing holiday meals, meeting clients for lunch, attending weddings and birthday parties, seeing a movie, and even going to a baseball game are all events where food plays a supporting, if not starring, role. You can learn to enjoy yourself at all these types of events *without* shifting fat burning into reverse. With the simple guidelines in this chapter, you will keep the weight coming off while living your life to the fullest. And after all, isn't that what this is all about?

Eating Out on the 1-Day Power Up

So what happens when your 1-Day Power Up falls on a day when you have to be out of town on a business trip? Or you're visiting your ailing grandma who has never even heard of protein powder? Or you'll be spending a good portion of the day at the airport? Don't worry. Sticking with your 1-Day Power Up when you're on the road is easier than you think. It just takes a bit of planning, preparation, and knowledge.

One of the best things you can do to keep from being caught unprepared on your 1-Day Power Up while on the road is to carry single-serving bags of protein powder and a fiber supplement—if you're using the Physicians Protein Smoothies Base Mix you won't need a separate fiber supplement because it's already included in the mix and packaged for a single serving—or keep a stash of your favorite flavors of the Physicians Protein Smoothies handy. You just need enough to get you through one day, so they won't take up much room in your purse, briefcase, or suitcase. And they're light so you won't be in danger of getting charged any excess baggage fees.

That way, when you get to Grandma's house, you can toss the protein powder into a blender with whatever fruit she has in the house and add a little bit of milk or even just water for a make-do smoothie. Or if you're using the Physicians Protein Smoothies, you just pick the flavor you want, add water, and shake—no blender necessary. It may not be as inventive as the smoothies you make at home, but it will do in a pinch to keep your metabolism fired up so you will lose weight overnight.

Tales of the Measuring Tape

"I went to visit my in-laws over the holidays so I took some protein powder with me for my 1-Day Power Up. They had frozen fruit in their freezer and skim milk in the fridge, so I just popped it all in their blender and voilà! It couldn't have been easier."
—Josh, 37, lost 26 pounds and is down from a size 38 to size 34 pants

---

What if you're nowhere near a blender and don't have your Physicians Protein Smoothies? Rest assured that smoothies have become so popular that whether you're in Peoria, Tuscaloosa, Albuquerque, or on the Hawaiian island of Maui, you can likely find a smoothie shop. You can find smoothie places in London, Japan, Korea, the Philippines, and even Dubai. Many airports boast smoothie vendors. And the fun, fruity concoctions are also popping up on menus at fast-food chains and coffee shops as well as in grocery store aisles.

But not all smoothies are created equal. The recipes here and the "Mix 'n' Match Smoothie Chart" have been carefully crafted—much work went into perfecting the combinations for maximum effect. Do you think the owners of your local "Smoothie Spot" have earned a medical degree, have helped thousands of people lose weight, have consulted with a registered dietitian, know how lean muscle affects weight loss, understand how protein is the building block for muscle, are aware of the dangers of the Shrinking Muscle Syndrome, or have analyzed the latest research on satiety? Probably not.

Some of their smoothies are fat-filled calorie hogs with virtually no protein or fiber. So they will pack on the pounds and still make you feel hungry sooner rather than later. Even that "Slim-Down Smoothie" that sounds so healthy might actually contribute to the Shrinking Muscle Syndrome and those abundant curvatures on your hips. So how can you decipher the menu so you know what to order?

Fortunately, most *do* have a few healthy options. You just have to be smart about how you order. In general, if you're looking for something that's going to prime your body for fat burning, keep it simple. The fewer the ingredients, the better. If you don't see anything on the menu that looks like it would earn 1-Day Power Up approval, don't be afraid to order off the menu. If you order a smoothie made with *only* the following ingredients, you should be in good shape—literally:

- Whey or soy protein—24–28 grams of protein
- Fiber—at least 5 grams
- Low-fat milk (1%), fat-free milk, soy milk, water, or ice
- Fresh or frozen fruit that isn't soaked in syrup
- Nonfat yogurt

To help make it easier for you, the nutritional data from some of the most popular smoothie chains, fast-food restaurants, coffee shops, and grocery store shelves has been examined, and in this chapter, you'll find the best options based on this analysis. When ordering or purchasing smoothies, make sure you get the serving sizes recommended here. And with some of them, you'll still need to add a protein boost or a fiber boost to make it worthy of the 1-Day Power Up. Some retailers offer nutritional boosts; others don't, so be sure you have your to-go bags of protein and fiber on you at all times.

Remember, these smoothies are for emergencies only. Don't make them a habit.

Smoothies on the Road

*Add protein boost (or multiple boosts) to get to 24–28 grams of protein.
**Add fiber boost (or multiple boosts) to get at least 5 grams of fiber.

Jamba Juice (all 16 ounces)

Nutritional Boosts:
Soy protein boost: 8 grams of protein
Whey protein boost: 10 grams of protein
Fiber boost: 7 grams of fiber

Flavor	Protein, grams	Fiber, grams
Berry Blend	11*	6
Peach Mango	11*	6
Strawberry Raspberry Banana	11*	7
Protein Berry Workout	17*	3**
Berry Fulfilling	6*	2**
Mango Mantra	7*	2**
Strawberry Nirvana	6*	2**

Robeks (all 12 ounces)

Nutritional Boosts:
Whey protein boost: 5 grams of protein
Soy protein boost: 6 grams of protein
Fiber boost: 5 grams of fiber

Flavor	Protein, grams	Fiber, grams
Pro Arobek	12*	2**
Cardio Cooler	9*	3**
Venice Burner	9*	3**

Smoothie King (all 20 ounces, ask to "Make It Skinny" to reduce sugar content and calories)

Nutritional Boosts:
Protein boost varies
Fiber boost: 8 grams of fiber

Flavor	Protein, grams	Fiber, grams
The Activator Chocolate	33	5
The Activator Vanilla	31	6
Gladiator	45	0**
High Protein Almond Mocha	30	2**
High Protein Banana	27	4**
High Protein Chocolate	30	2**
High Protein Lemon	26	1**
High Protein Pineapple	28	2**
Lean1 Chocolate	22*	7
Lean1 Strawberry	20*	5
Lean1 Vanilla	22*	5
The Shredder—Chocolate	39	1**
The Shredder—Strawberry	30	3**
The Shredder—Vanilla	36	0**

Planet Smoothie (all 22 ounces, includes protein boost)

Nutritional Boosts:
Whey protein boost: 6 grams of protein
Fiber boost: 2 grams of fiber

Flavor	Protein, grams	Fiber, grams
Big Bang	13*	5
Chocolate Chimp	15*	5
Mr. Mongo Chocolate	20*	11
Planet Pro Light	26	7

Orange Julius (serving sizes vary, see chart)

Nutritional Boosts:
Protein boost: 7 grams of protein
Fiber boost: 6 grams of fiber

Flavor	Protein, grams	Fiber, grams
Strawberry Delight (32 oz.)	3*	5
Berry Pom Twilight (32 oz.)	3*	6
Pineapple Daylight (32 oz.)	2*	4**
Tropical Sunlight (32 oz.)	3*	3**
Berry Banana Squeeze (20 oz.)	1*	4**
Blackberry Storm (12 oz.)	6*	3**
Blackberry Toner (20 oz.)	7*	4**
Cocoa Latte Swirl (16 oz.)	9*	2**
Mango Passion (20 oz.)	7*	2**
Pomegranate & Berries (20 oz.)	7*	3**
Raspberry Crème (12 oz.)	6*	2**
Raspberry Crush (20 oz.)	2*	7
Strawberry Xtreme (20 oz.)	7*	3**
Tropical Tango (20 oz.)	1*	3**

Starbucks (all 16 ounces with nonfat milk)
Nutritional Boosts: None, bring your own!

Flavor	Protein, grams	Fiber, grams
Chocolate Smoothie	20*	7
Strawberry Smoothie	16*	7

Jack-in-the-Box (all 16 ounces)
Nutritional Boosts: None, bring your own!

Flavor	Protein, grams	Fiber, grams
Strawberry Smoothie	2*	1**
Strawberry Banana Smoothie	2*	1**

McDonald's (all 22 ounces)
Nutritional Boosts: None, bring your own!

Flavor	Protein, grams	Fiber, grams
Strawberry Banana Smoothie	3*	4**
Wild Berry Smoothie	3*	4**
Mango Pineapple Smoothie	4*	3**

Subway (all 15 ounces)
Nutritional Boosts: None, bring your own!

Flavor	Protein, grams	Fiber, grams
Mango Smoothie	6*	0**
Strawberry Smoothie	6*	0**

Store-Bought Smoothies (serving sizes vary, see chart)
Nutritional Boosts: None, bring your own!

Flavor	Protein, grams	Fiber, grams
Physicians Protein Smoothies: Chocolate Peanut Butter Cup (8 oz.)	40	5
Physicians Protein Smoothies: California Dreaming (8 oz.)	40	5
Physicians Protein Smoothies: Super Green Machine (8 oz.)	40	5
Naked Apple Raisin Oat (9.5 oz.)	13*	5
Naked Blueberry Oat (9.5 oz.)	12*	5
Naked Peach Mango Oat (9.5 oz.)	12*	5
Sunkist Naturals Orange Cream (12 oz.)	19*	0**
Sunkist Naturals Berries & Cream (12 oz.)	19*	0**
Sunkist Naturals Piña Colada (12 oz.)	19*	2**
Lifeway Low-fat Kefir—any flavor (8 oz.)—it's okay to get 2	11*	0**
Evolution Fresh Protein Power (15.2 oz.)	26	0**

Tales of the Measuring Tape

"I used to order this smoothie that I thought was going to help me lose weight, but after I learned what to look for in a smoothie, I realized that the one I was drinking didn't have any protein and had virtually no fiber. It was basically calories and sugar. No wonder I always felt so hungry right after I drank it. Now when I'm traveling, I know which smoothies to order and when I need to add a protein boost. And I can go for hours afterward without my stomach growling."

—Nikki, 24, lost 16 pounds

Eating Out on the 6-Day Fuel Up

So you've cleaned all the junk food out of your cupboards and filled your kitchen with good-for-you fruits, vegetables, lean carbs, lean protein, and healthy fats. You're eating a delicious, protein-packed, high-fiber lunch that keeps you satisfied all afternoon—no more vending machine calling your name at three o'clock. You're whipping up 15-minute and no-cook recipes at home and loving them. And even better, your pants are feeling looser and your arms don't jiggle the way they used to. Way to go!

Now your coworkers have just invited you out to lunch to celebrate your office mate's birthday. What do you do? You know that many restaurants use cooking techniques and ingredients that are loaded with saturated fats, refined carbohydrates, sugar, and salt, and that the portion sizes are often way out of control. All of these can be a recipe for weight gain, bloating, and fat production. Should you just say no thanks and hide in your office while you eat the food you brought from home? There's no need to panic or shrink like a wallflower. Take a deep breath, arm yourself with the following tips, and have a great time!

These simple strategies worked for Angela, who was almost 50 pounds overweight when she showed up at the Nutrition and Weight Management Center at Boston Medical Center. She had tried to lose weight, but whenever she and her friends would go out to eat, it turned into a free-for-all. She would always tell herself she wasn't going to overeat, but as soon as the server put the basket of bread or the chips and salsa on the table, she would dig in, and her resolve would quickly evaporate. Then when she opened the menu, her eyes would dart quickly from one diet disaster to the next—bacon cheeseburger with fries, fettuccini Alfredo, chicken potpie. Sometimes she would give in and order the calorie bomb.

Other times she would choose something that she thought sounded healthy but then turned out to be full of fat and calories. For example, one time she ordered a salad with peaches and crispy chicken. She thought to herself, "It's peaches with chicken—it must be healthy. And it's just a salad so I'll go ahead and get the full order instead of the half." Wrong! Here's what was in that seemingly innocent salad:

1,200 calories
20 grams of saturated fat

Yes, it did have ample amounts of protein and fiber, but it was big enough for three people to share. The list of ingredients offered clues that could have tipped her off to the high calorie count:

- **Caramelized peaches:** "Caramelized" means it's made with gobs of butter and sugar.
- **Dried cranberries:** Dried fruits like cranberries are often full of extra sugar in the coating.
- **Caramelized pecans:** More butter and sugar.
- **Feta cheese**: Probably full-fat.
- **Crispy breaded chicken:** "Crispy" is a code word for "fried" and foods are typically breaded with some form of refined flour.
- **Blue cheese dressing:** One of the fattiest, highest-calorie dressings around.

On that particular day, Angela also downed two strawberry lemonades and decided that since she had only had a salad, she would split a dessert with her friends. They wanted to keep it simple so they opted for a slice of butter cake à la mode. That added 1,400 calories and nearly 60 grams of saturated fat! Even divided by the three of them, it was still more than 450 calories apiece. Angela left the restaurant that day feeling bloated. By that evening, she figured she had already blown her diet so she ordered a pizza for dinner and had a pint of Häagen-Dazs Dulce de Leche ice cream for dessert.

Angela needed some tips to help her make better choices when eating out. Here's what she learned.

Order off the Menu

Most restaurants these days are very accommodating and will eagerly make substitutions. In fact, you don't even have to bother looking at the menu. You could just ask for the following:

- Grilled chicken breast or grilled, baked, or poached fish— plain, without any butter or sauce
- Steamed vegetables
- Quinoa, brown rice, or whole-wheat pasta
- 1 glass of wine

Many restaurants will accommodate you. If a restaurant doesn't have any brown rice, quinoa, or whole-wheat pasta, you can always double or even triple up on the vegetables. They may charge a little bit extra when you do this, but isn't it worth a few dollars to keep the fat coming off and to boost your health while you're at it?

Know Before You Go

Thanks to the Internet, it's easier than ever to check out the nutritional info at restaurants before you sit down to peruse the menu. Whenever possible, choose your entrée before you get to the restaurant. And then don't even open your menu at the table. Tune out when the server tells you about their "amazing" specials and order first so you aren't tempted by anyone else's order. Stick to the smart choice.

Decode the Menu

Decrypting a menu is similar to translating a foreign language. Those ingenious restaurant marketing gurus slip in words that make some foods sound healthy when they really aren't. And sometimes the same culinary term might indicate a dish that gets the green light or one that you should skip. For example, baked fish gets a thumbs-up, but baked cookies don't. A crisp pear salad can be a good choice, but an apple crisp isn't. Clearly, it can get a bit confusing.

Knowing how to translate those culinary clichés will help you get an A+ in healthy ordering. You may want to keep the following lists with you as a sort of cheat sheet when dining out so you can translate those menus and stay on track. The "Green Light" terms are the ones that are likely to help you keep the weight coming off. The "Yellow Light" terms are a little trickier because they may denote a healthy option in some cases but not in others. Check out the descriptions of these terms for clarification. The "Red Light" terms typically indicate menu choices that slow your fat-burning engines and are more likely to pad your hips and thighs.

Green Light

Boiled	Roasted
Grilled	Steamed
Poached	Whole Grain

Yellow Light

Baked	Multigrain
Broiled/Charbroiled	Organic
Crisp/Crispy	Sautéed
Crunchy	Seasoned

Fat-Free   Spiced/Spicy
Fresh   Stir-Fried
Garnish   Vegetarian
Light/Lite   Vinaigrette
Marinated

Yellow Light Terms Decoded

Baked: Baked poultry and fish are great, but baked cookies and muffins aren't.

Broiled/Charbroiled: This means being cooked over intense heat. The cooking method is fine, as long as there's no butter, but it also depends on what is being broiled—a half-pound burger or a few shrimp?

Crisp/Crispy: Crisp lettuce is good, but apple crisp, crispy coated chicken breast, and crispy onion rings aren't.

Crunchy: Crunchy vegetables get a thumbs-up, but crunchy tortilla chips in your salad don't.

Fat-Free: Don't be fooled by the fat-free tag—just because it's fat-free doesn't mean you can order two or three. Many fat-free products have a higher sugar content.

Fresh: Fresh tomatoes and other vegetables are great, but fresh-baked pastries and fresh cheese may not help you reach your goal weight.

Garnish: If it's garnished with a parsley sprig, okay. If it's garnished with sour cream, garlic mayo, or some other fattening sauce, say no thanks.

Light/Lite: Light variations of meals may have fewer calories but may have also been stripped of fiber and protein.

Marinated: Find out what it's marinated in—a sugary glaze (no thanks!) or red wine vinegar (okay)? As a rule, look for marinades that are low in fat and sugar.

Multigrain: Multigrain is not always whole grain; don't take a chance.

Organic: How can something organic be bad for your diet? When it's fried, breaded, or smothered in cream sauce.

Sautéed: Sautéed means that something is fried quickly. Ask for it to be sautéed in a small amount of oil or use cooking spray instead.

Seasoned: Being seasoned with herbs is ideal, but watch out if butter or oil is thrown into the mix.

Spiced/Spicy: Spices are a wonderful way to add flavor or a little kick. It's too bad restaurants also often add butter, fat, or cream to these spices. Ask how the dish is prepared.

Stir-Fried: This basically means fried quickly. Ask for your food to be stir-fried in a small amount of oil or use cooking spray instead.

Vegetarian: Just because something is meatless doesn't necessarily make it healthy. Vegetarian lasagna can be a cheesy mess that will slow down your metabolism, so be aware.

Vinaigrette: Vinaigrette is a good choice for salad dressing, but many places use far too much of it. Always ask for it on the side.

Red Light

Au gratin	Crumb-Coated
Basted	Crust/Crusted
Battered	Dip/Dipping Sauce
Breaded	Fried/Deep-Fried/
Buttered/Butter Sauce	Flash-Fried/Pan-
Candied	Fried
Caramelized	Glazed
Cheesy	Herb-Crusted
Coated	Melted
Country-Style	Stuffed
Creamy/Creamed/	Tempura
Cream Sauce	

Ethnic Dining

Not every restaurant prepares meals the same way, but there are some general guidelines you can follow at your favorite ethnic restaurant.

Chinese

Consider: Appetizers with lettuce wraps • Steamed dumplings • Szechwan dishes with sauces made from chicken stock, such as garlic sauce • Whole steamed fish for sharing • Steamed meats and vegetables

Pass on: Fried rice • Fried wontons and spring rolls • Moo shu pork • Sweet-and-sour dishes • Duck • Nut dishes

French

Consider: Broth-based stews such as bouillabaisse • Coq au vin • Salade niçoise

Pass on: Au gratin dishes, which are made with cheese, butter, and sometimes cream • Hollandaise or béarnaise sauces • Dessert pastries • Quiches • Pâté

Greek

Consider: Fish baked with garlic and tomato-based plaki sauce • Shish kabob or any grilled lamb dish • Torato

Pass on: Avgolemono • Baklava • Moussaka • Falafel • Kibbeh

Italian

Consider: Florentine dishes, usually chicken or veal dressed with spinach • Pastas with tomato-based sauces • Primavera pasta • Clam sauce • Mussels • Polenta • Pizza (one thin slice with oil blotted and topped with vegetables)

Pass on: Alfredo dishes • Pasta carbonara • Pizza topped with sausage, pepperoni, or other meats • Pesto sauce

Japanese

Consider: Miso soup • Sukiyaki • Fish and vegetable sushi and sashimi • Teriyaki (chicken, fish, and beef)

Pass on: Anything "crispy" • Fried meat • Tempura

Mexican

Consider: Chicken enchiladas or burritos without cheese • Salsas served with baked chips • Seviche • Soft tacos • Veracruz dishes, which are made from tomatoes, onions, and chilis

Pass on: Anything made with sour cream and cheese • Fried chips and taco shells • Refried beans • Chorizo

Middle Eastern
Consider: Anything made with couscous or tabbouleh • Lavash • Lentil dishes • Moroccan stew • Baba ghanoush and hummus spreads
Pass on: Dips floating in oil • Falafel • Stuffed grape leaves, which usually come bathed in oil

Thai
Consider: Chicken satay (dip into the peanut sauce sparingly) • Hot and spicy soups • Noodle bowls • Steamed or grilled fish
Pass on: Coconut curries • Pad thai

Pay Attention to Portions

In America, we've got a serious case of portion distortion. Restaurants serve massive plates piled high with food. And if your mom taught you to "clean your plate," you probably think you're supposed to eat everything they serve. It's time for you to take control of the portions you eat. Some restaurants offer half portions, and even if you don't see it listed on the menu, ask if you can get a half portion. You can also split an entrée with a friend or spouse or ask the server to put half of your meal in a to-go container *before* bringing it to your table. To avoid ending up with a jumbo meal, avoid ordering menu items that use these terms.

- *Combo:* This usually indicates two meals in one, like steak and fish or eggs and pancakes.
- *Generous:* "Generous" portions will generate more fat cells.
- *Monster:* Anything that's "monster" sized will increase your size.
- *Value:* Is it really a value meal if it makes you gain weight and harms your health?

On her next appointment, Angela shared her latest restaurant experience. Once again, her friends asked her to go out for lunch. This time, she jumped online to look at the restaurant's menu first. Based on the nutritional info, she decided on a roasted vegetable salad with grilled chicken—a half order, which most restaurants offer at lunch. You can typically order a lunch-sized portion at dinner, too. You just need to ask.

When they got to the restaurant, Angela asked the server to take the bread away from the table after her friends had taken their share from the bread basket. She ordered first so she wouldn't be influenced by what her friends were ordering. She asked for fat-free vinaigrette on the side and only used about half of it. She stuck to water with her meal, and when her friends mentioned dessert, Angela opted for a decaf iced cappuccino that came in under 100 calories. Altogether, she shaved off almost 2,000 calories from her lunchtime meal. She left feeling pleasantly full and, best of all, good about her decisions. Later that night, she ate reasonably and woke up 1 pound lighter the next day.

What Angela realized is that with a few small tweaks, she could go out with her friends and still eat a healthy meal that tasted great but would also help her lose weight. You can, too, if you follow these guidelines.

Restaurant Meals—From Bad to Better

A single restaurant meal can do a lot of damage and can shift your body from burning fat to storing it. There are many dishes that certainly won't do your body any favors, and you should beware of restaurants that don't provide nutritional info. But there are restaurant meals, and even some fast-food meals, that will help you maintain the metabolic marvel you achieve on this diet. Here is what to order at some of the most popular chain restaurants.

Restaurant Meals—What to Order

Au Bon Pain	Turkey, Apple, Brie, and Spinach Salad w/fat-free Raspberry Vinaigrette
Baja Fresh	2 Original Baja Tacos (chicken)
Burger King	Tendergrill Garden Salad w/Ken's Light Italian dressing
Chili's	Classic Sirloin, House Salad w/fat-free Honey Mustard dressing
California Pizza Kitchen	Half Roasted Vegetable Salad w/grilled shrimp w/fat-free vinaigrette, Kids Fresh Fruit
Dairy Queen	Grilled Chicken Salad w/fat-free dressing *or* Grilled Chicken Sandwich *or* Grilled Chicken Wrap; Vanilla Cream Bar *or* Fudge Bar
Denny's	"Build Your Own Grand Slam"—2 egg whites, turkey bacon strips, oatmeal, seasonal fruit
Dunkin' Donuts	Egg White Veggie Wake-Up, plain Oatmeal w/Dried Fruit Topping
Golden Corral	Baked New Orleans Style Fish (2 pieces) *or* Chicken Breast (2 pieces) *or* Turkey Breast w/Wing; green beans, tomatoes and okra, Key West Vegetable Blend
IHOP	Simple & Fit—Two Egg Breakfast (scrambled egg substitute), 2 strips turkey bacon, whole-wheat toast, seasonal fresh fruit
LongHorn Steakhouse	Grilled Fresh Rainbow Trout *or* LongHorn Salmon (7 oz.), Fresh Seasonal Vegetables, Mixed Green Side Salad w/fat-free Ranch
McDonald's	Premium Grilled Chicken Classic Sandwich, Side Salad, Apple Slices
Olive Garden	Minestrone Soup, Venetian Apricot Chicken
Outback Steakhouse	Victoria's Filet (6 oz., no topping), Fresh Seasonal Mixed Vegetables, grilled asparagus, green beans
Panera Bread	Half Smoked Turkey Breast Sandwich on Whole Wheat, Low-Fat Garden Vegetable Soup w/Pesto
P.F. Chang's	Shrimp Dumplings (steamed), spinach stir-fried w/garlic, brown rice
Pizza Hut	1 slice Fit 'n' Delicious Chicken, Mushroom & Jalapeño Pizza

continued

Restaurant Meals—What to Order (continued)

Red Lobster	Half Portion Rainbow Trout, broccoli, Garden Salad w/Petite Shrimp Salad Topping
Ruby Tuesday	Petite Creole Catch, grilled zucchini, steamed broccoli, sliced tomatoes w/vinaigrette
Starbucks	Turkey Bacon & White Cheddar Classic Breakfast Sandwich
Subway	6" Roast Beef *or* Ham *or* Turkey *or* Oven Roasted Chicken sandwich; Tomato Garden Vegetable w/Rotini, Apple Slices
Taco Bell	2 Fresco Chicken Soft Tacos
Uno Chicago Grill	Steak Marsala, Farro Salad, Veggie Soup
Wendy's	Grilled Chicken Go Wrap, Garden Side Salad, Apple Slices

Holidays

Happy holidays! Did you know that your friends, family, coworkers, and employers are all chipping in to get you something? Do you want to know what it is? A spare tire. Yes, all those well-meaning folks with their holiday meals, parties, cocktails, and treats conspire to slow your metabolism to a screeching halt and cause your fat cells to start expanding like party balloons. The Overnight Diet is designed to help you combat typical holiday weight gain. The 6-Day Fuel Up keeps hunger at bay and makes you less likely to experience intense cravings for fattening holiday fare. And even if you overindulge at a holiday event, the 1-Day Power Up can help put you back on track. Here are some surefire strategies to help you muscle through the holiday season so you can keep the weight coming off:

Eat before you go. Have a healthy, high-protein, high-fiber snack or small meal before that holiday party or celebration meal. The protein and fiber will ensure that you won't be starving and tempted to grab every appetizer that comes your way. Don't have time for a meal with protein and fiber? Eat an apple on your way to the party. It can curb your appetite.

Get the Skinny on the Science

An Apple on the Way Saves the Day Eating an apple fifteen minutes prior to a meal reduces intake at that meal by 15 percent, according to a study in *Appetite* from researchers at Penn State. This trial, which involved 30 men and 28 women, also showed that eating a whole apple caused a greater reduction in subsequent intake than having applesauce or apple juice with added fiber.

Go for the 6-Day Fuel Up–friendly foods first. As soon as you arrive, search for any raw vegetables or fruit, lean protein such as shrimp, or whole-grain crackers, and take a small plate of them. Noshing on these foods will keep your mouth occupied and increase satiety so you are less likely to overindulge on the fattier fare.

Scout out the buffet, then choose. With buffet-style meals, don't load up your plate as you go through the line. Scan all the offerings first, then take only the few things that you really love.

Don't park yourself next to the buffet. Take the advice of Brian Wansink, a Cornell University professor and author of *Mindless Eating*, and sit as far away from the buffet as you can while you eat.

BYOD. Bring your own dish, if it's okay with your hosts. Chicken and veggie skewers or a spinach salad with turkey breast are good options that can look festive, plus you can make an entire meal out of them.

Get back on track. So you overdid it at the office shindig. Don't beat yourself up about it. Just get back to the 1-Day Power Up or 6-Day Fuel Up, depending on the day of the week.

Vacations

Just because you're going on vacation doesn't mean you have to take a vacation from your healthy eating habits. Whether you're hitting the slopes, sinking your toes in the sand, or hopping aboard a cruise ship for a little R&R, you can certainly find options that will keep the scale going in the right direction. Here are a few tips to remember:

Have it your way. Whether you're ordering room service or dining at a resort, don't be shy about asking for substitutions—fruit instead of French fries, broccoli instead of onion rings, white meat instead of dark meat chicken, whole-wheat instead of white bread.

Zero in on healthy options. If you're vacationing on an all-inclusive cruise or resort, you will likely be faced with an endless buffet of fattening foods and beverages morning, noon, and night—not to mention midmorning, afternoon, and late at night. Use the tips provided earlier on mastering holiday buffets to help you find the best choices amid the dizzying array of calorie bombs.

Keep up with the Quickie Rev Up. The Quickie Rev Up was designed specifically so you can do it anywhere, anytime. You don't need any equipment, so you can do it in your hotel room, on a sandy beach, or on a cruise ship deck.

Take Me Out to the Ball Game

The Nutrition and Weight Management Center at Boston Medical Center just happens to be located in one of the greatest sports towns in the world. In Boston, people take baseball, basketball, football, and hockey seriously, and there's nothing better than going to a game. But inside the hallowed halls of these ballparks and arenas lurk some of the most fattening food concoctions you will ever find.

What's even worse is that more ballparks are offering All You Can Eat seats, sections where an additional fee will get you an unlimited supply of hot dogs, peanuts, and Cracker Jack. Believe me, that's a

Ballpark Foods	Size (approx.)	Calories
Hot Dog	Foot-long	400+
Peanuts	12 oz.	1,200+
Cracker Jack	Stadium size	400+
Nachos with Cheese	12 oz.	1,500+
Soft Pretzel	7–8 oz.	700+

Sources: SportsIllustrated.com, KCBY.com

bottomless buffet you do *not* want to take part in. The table opposite gives a peek at the damage you can do with some ballpark favorites.

Take heart. Going to a game doesn't have to go hand in hand with a food binge. In fact, many of the nation's ballparks are adding healthy options to their menus. It's not uncommon to find turkey dogs, turkey sandwiches on whole wheat, veggie burgers and "not" dogs, salads, sushi, raw veggies, fresh produce, and fruit and yogurt parfaits. Choose wisely or eat before you go.

At the Movies

For some people, the movie theater is where they are most tempted to stray from their new healthy eating habits. It's easy to see why. As soon as you step into the theater lobby, your senses are assaulted by the smell of popcorn wafting through the air. But beware of those snacks at the concession stand. They are packed with fat, grease, and calories. In fact, a medium-sized popcorn from the nation's largest theater chain has as many calories as a Big Mac, large fries, and a medium Coke from McDonald's! Take a look at the calorie counts for some of the most popular movie snacks. This might scare you more than the latest horror flick!

Movie Snacks	*Size*	*Calories*	*Sat Fat*
Popcorn	Medium (20 cups)	1,200	60g
Twizzlers	5 oz.	460	0g
Skittles, Original	4 oz.	450	4g
Junior Mints, XL	4.8 oz.	570	8g
Raisinets	3.5 oz.	420	11g
M&M's, Milk Chocolate	3.4 oz	480	11g
Goobers	3.5 oz.	510	12g
M&M's, Peanut	5.3 oz.	790	16g
Reese's Pieces	8 oz.	1,160	35g
Nachos	about 40 chips	1,100	18.5g
Soda	54 oz.	500	0

Sources: Center for Science in the Public Interest, Moviefone.com

Our nation's theaters have been slow to offer healthy alternatives, but that may be changing. At the 2010 convention of movie theater owners, it was reported that two-thirds of moviegoers surveyed would buy healthier concessions if they were available. However, until your local theater is stocked with fresh fruit, turkey sandwiches on whole-grain bread, and chicken skewers, bring your own snacks!

As you can see, it is up to you to take charge of what you consume. Don't let a bunch of profit-hungry restaurant, hotel, ballpark, and movie theater marketing gurus tell you what to eat. You tell them what you want. Your body will thank you for it.

CHAPTER 11

I Reached My Goal Weight...
Now What?

You've made it! After all that time battling your weight, you're finally seeing that magic number on your scale. Even more exciting, your body isn't just a slimmed-down version of your fatter self. It has been completely resculpted, as if someone chiseled away at it to give your arms, abs, hips, thighs, and back end more definition. Those long, lean muscles you've developed have given you a sleeker figure than you ever imagined. You actually get a kick out of shopping for clothes now because everything fits you better. On top of that, you're bursting with energy. What could be better? Maintaining that toned new shape and vitality for decades to come, that's what.

Losing weight is only half the battle. Keeping it off can be an even tougher challenge. Many people can lose weight—numerous times for some of them—but they haven't found a way to maintain their new smaller size. That's what happened to Rhonda. She went on a fad crash diet and lost some weight. But when she finished the diet, she went right back to the way she was eating before. It's no surprise Rhonda quickly ballooned up to her former shape. When Rhonda went on the Overnight Diet, she wanted to know if it would be any different. Yes, Rhonda, it is.

The Overnight Diet for Life

Helping you get to your goal weight quickly is only the first part of this diet. Just as much time has been devoted to engineering a post-diet plan to help you maintain that weight loss for the long term. The Overnight Diet for Life is that plan, and it is designed to maintain the powerful synergy you achieved from this combo diet. By following the Overnight Diet for Life guidelines, you will:

- Maintain your new cinched-in waistline.
- Preserve the lean muscle you have developed.
- Keep your metabolism running at lightning-fast speed.
- Keep your fat genes in the "off" mode.
- Continue to enjoy greater energy.
- Keep water retention and bloating at bay.
- Keep inflammation under control.
- Maintain enhanced insulin sensitivity.
- Minimize your risk for disease.

And the best part is that you can do all this while enjoying an even greater variety of foods.

Tales of the Measuring Tape

"I had lost and regained about 20 to 30 pounds at least five times in my lifetime, so I was afraid that I would gain the weight back again this time, too. Thank goodness the Overnight Diet comes with a plan on how to keep the weight off once you lose it. I've kept my new weight for three years, and counting!"

—Sasha, 43, lost 30 pounds

Following the Overnight Diet for Life is easy. Just continue to alternate between the 1-Day Power Up and the 6-Day Fuel Up—with a few very important modification rules.

Rule 1: Modify the 1-Day Power Up to fit your individual needs.

The 1-Day Power Up continues to play an important role in maintaining your new physique, but you can modify it depending on your needs and goals. Here are three ways to change up your smoothie feast day and still keep the weight off.

Add whole-food snacks. Continue to have three jumbo smoothies on the 1-Day Power Up but add in two to three small whole-food snacks, such as raw veggies and dip, fruit, string cheese wrapped in a slice of turkey, or nonfat yogurt. Mariana, fifty-four, who lost 36 pounds on the diet, has kept them off for almost five years this way. She has a smoothie for breakfast, a piece of fruit, a smoothie for lunch, sliced red bell pepper and a piece of fat-free cheese, a smoothie for dinner, and then a fat-free yogurt with berries.

Swap one smoothie for a whole meal. Switch to having two smoothies a day and one whole meal. It's up to you which meal you prefer—breakfast, lunch, or dinner. Thirty-three-year-old Katrina has been following this plan for more than two years since she lost 18 pounds and hasn't gained back a single pound. She likes to blend up a smoothie for breakfast, eats a full lunch, then sips on another smoothie for dinner. But if she has a business dinner or a night out with friends on her 1-Day Power Up, she simply enjoys smoothies for both breakfast and lunch instead.

Tales of the Measuring Tape

"Keeping the weight off has been so easy. I love that the 1-Day Power Up can be so flexible. I always find a way to make it work with my schedule."

—Katrina, 33, lost 18 pounds

Swap two smoothies for whole meals. You may find that having just one smoothie along with two solid meals on your 1-Day Power Up will continue to keep you in shape. This combo has been working for thirty-year-old Joshua, who shed 25 pounds more than three and a half years ago. He starts his 1-Day Power Up with an invigo-rating smoothie, then typically has a lunch and a dinner from the 6-Day Fuel Up recipes.

Which option is right for you? After you reach your goal weight, it's best to either add in a few whole-food snacks or swap one smoothie for a whole meal. If you continue to lose weight with either of these options, then shift to having two whole-food meals and just one smoothie on your 1-Day Power Up.

Take note that some people find that they really love the way they feel on their smoothie day and want to continue getting the many health benefits a liquid feast day provides. For this reason, they keep following the basic 1-Day Power Up—with three jumbo smoothies a day—long after they have reached their goal weight.

At age forty-six, Lorraine wanted to shed the 20 pounds of excess baggage she had been lugging around since her college days. At first, she was very hesitant to try the 1-Day Power Up and was afraid she would be starving and exhausted all day long. Instead, she found that she felt especially energized on her smoothie day and couldn't be happier that she didn't have to do any cooking on that day. Plus, she loved the idea that she was doing something good for her health. So when Lorraine succeeded in losing those 20 pounds, she didn't want to give up her smoothie day. That was almost five years ago, and now at age fifty-one she is still doing a weekly smoothie day and loving it. She makes sure to eat enough on the other six days of the week to maintain her weight and feels great.

This is very important: If you ever find yourself gaining a few pounds—say you've overindulged during the holidays or on a vacation—go back to square one. Revert back to the basic 1-Day Power Up, to reignite fat burning and rapid weight loss, and stick to the basic 6-Day Fuel Up, alternating from one to the other until you get back down to your goal weight.

Rule 2: Tweak the 6-Day Fuel Up for a greater variety of foods.

As you transition to the Overnight Diet for Life phase, you will need to make a few modifications to the 6-Day Fuel Up. But that's not a bad thing! You will get to eat an even greater variety of foods that will fill you up and keep you satisfied. I'm talking about adding in more starchy vegetables such as potatoes and yams, increasing the number of servings of whole grains you consume, and being a little more generous with those healthy fats. Here's how to tweak the 6-Day Fuel Up.

Keep meeting your DPR every day for life. It is essential that you continue to fuel up on 1.5 grams of lean protein per kilogram of ideal body weight per day. At this point, though, your ideal weight is probably a lot closer to your actual weight. Adequate intake of protein is a big part of what helped you lose the fat and develop lean muscle, and it plays an integral role in allowing you to maintain your new shape. Keep your protein intake at this level throughout the remainder of your life, regardless of your age. As we discussed, getting the right amount and the right kind of protein fuels muscles and boosts metabolism. It also ranks high in terms of satiety, so it keeps you feeling full, which is critical to maintaining weight loss.

Enjoy more starchy vegetables. Love potatoes or yams? Feel free to increase your consumption of starchy vegetables up to 2 cups per day. Starchy vegetables include corn, parsnips, potatoes, sweet potatoes, winter squash, peas, pumpkin, yams, and yucca. This doesn't mean you can load up your plate with a mound of French fries; that isn't going to help you maintain your weight. But savoring half a baked potato, half a cup of peas or corn, or a few baked sweet potato fries with a meal can satisfy your taste buds and keep your waistline under control. Pay attention to preparation, too. Good bets include baking, steaming, roasting, and boiling.

Eat an extra 1–2 servings of whole grains per day. Bread lovers and pasta lovers, rejoice! I'm giving you permission to eat more of the doughy goodness you love. Just make sure you stick to whole grains rather than refined carbs and watch your portion sizes. One serving means one slice of whole-grain bread, one cup of 100 percent whole-grain cereal, or half a cup of cooked brown rice—*not* one Krispy Kreme doughnut.

Enjoy an extra drizzle of healthy fat. Continue to make healthy PUFAs and MUFAs the main fats in your diet, but feel free to add an extra drizzle, spray, or dollop to your meals. This goes for nuts, seeds, and avocados, too. But don't go crazy dipping your additional servings of whole-grain bread into a bucket of olive oil. Moderation is always essential.

Keep drinking at least 8 cups of fluids a day and continue savoring a daily glass of wine if you like. Staying adequately hydrated juices up your metabolism for the long haul. That's why it's important to continue drinking at least 8 cups of fluids a day. You also get to continue enjoying a nightly glass of wine. Your best bet is to stick with the approved 6-Day Fuel Up fluids for good because so many regular sodas, coffee concoctions, fruit juices, cocktails, and energy drinks are loaded with sugar, fat, and calories, which slow metabolism.

Rule 3: When the Quickie Rev Up starts feeling too easy, ramp up the intensity.

When you do the Quickie Rev Up on a regular basis, you will find that moves that seemed really challenging at first start to feel easier. You can do more reps or you can do the reps faster than when you first started. While you may like the fact that your workout has gotten easier, your muscles don't. Keeping your muscles challenged is the key to maintaining lean muscle mass. When exercises become too easy for you, switch to the more advanced body-weight moves or try higher-intensity Rev Up Blasts. You'll be ready for it. And if those become too easy, there are many ways to increase the challenge, including using machines at a gym, free weights, kettle bells, or medicine balls.

Let Me Help You Keep It Off

In this book, I've given you the guidelines you need to lose 5, 15, or 50-plus pounds and keep them off. I've tried to make this diet as easy as possible to follow, but I know that you may have some questions I didn't anticipate. That's why I have created a website (OvernightDiet.org) where you can go for additional advice, smoothie-making tips, exercise demonstrations (you might even see *me* demonstrating some of them!), and more. You can also find motivational tips and favorite recipes from other dieters who have already lost the weight or who are on their journey to lasting weight loss just like you. I want to hear from you, too, so feel free to share your success, your insights on what's working for you, or your latest sinlessly delicious smoothie creation. This website is like having me as your very own diet doctor guiding you through the weight-loss process so you can look better, feel better, and live longer. Let's do this together.

Appendix A

1-Day Power Up Toolkit

Here, you will find helpful tools to create your own 1-Day Power Up smoothies. Discover just some of the amazing flavorings, extracts, and spices that can add a powerful punch of taste to your smoothies. And use the step-by-step "Mix 'n' Match Smoothie Chart" to make your own smoothie creations. You'll find a shopping list that includes ingredients for the 1-Day Power Up in Appendix B.

Mix 'n' Match Smoothie Chart

Protein (choose 1)	1 scoop protein powder, Physicians Protein Smoothies Base Mix, whey, or soy
	1 cup fat-free Greek yogurt
Liquid (choose 1)	½ cup fat-free milk
	½ cup light soy milk
	1 cup almond milk, unsweetened
	¼ cup light coconut milk, unsweetened
	½ cup coconut water, unsweetened
	¼ cup juice of your choice
Fruits (choose up to 2)	½ apple, medium
	½ banana, medium
	½ cup blueberries
	¼ cup cherries, pitted
	½ cup grapes, seedless

continued

Mix 'n' Match Smoothie Chart (continued)

Fruits (continued) *(choose up to 2)*	1 kiwi 1 lemon 1 lime ½ cup mango 1 nectarine, small pitted 1 orange, small ½ cup papaya ½ cup peaches ½ pear, medium ½ cup pineapple 1 plum, pitted ½ cup raspberries ½ cup sliced strawberries
Veggies *(choose up to 3)*	1 cup arugula 1 carrot, small 1 celery stalk, medium ½ cup sliced cucumber ½ cup chopped fresh kale ½ cup mint leaves 1 cup fresh romaine lettuce 1 cup fresh Swiss chard 1 cup fresh spinach 1 tomato, small
Add-Ins *(optional,* *choose up to 2)*	1 teaspoon agave nectar 1 tablespoon avocado 1 teaspoon blackstrap molasses 1 teaspoon chocolate syrup, fat-free 1 tablespoon cocoa powder, unsweetened 1 stick pack CocoaVia supplement 1 teaspoon creamy peanut butter 1 tablespoon oats, dry, old-fashioned 1 teaspoon seeds (flaxseeds, pumpkin, sunflower)

Freebies (optional, choose 1)	½ cup brewed coffee
	1 flavoring/extract of your choice, as directed, up to 1 teaspoon
	½ cup brewed green tea
	¼–½ teaspoon spice of your choice
	Ice—more ice makes smoothie thicker
	Salt and pepper to taste
	1 serving Truvia or Splenda
	Water—more water makes smoothie thinner

Smoothie Flavorings and Extracts

Amaretto	Coconut	Pecan
Anise	Coffee	Peppermint
Banana cream	Cotton candy	Piña colada
Butter rum	Eggnog	Pound cake
Butterscotch	English toffee	Pralines 'n' cream
Caramel	Hazelnut	Pumpkin
Champagne	Marshmallow	Root beer
Cheesecake	Peanut butter	

Smoothie Spices

Allspice	Jalapeño
Anise	Nutmeg
Cinnamon	Orange peel
Cloves	Parsley
Coriander	Pumpkin pie spice
Ginger	Wasabi powder

Appendix B

6-Day Fuel Up Toolkit

To help you prepare for the 6-Day Fuel Up as well as the 1-Day Power Up, use the "Overnight Diet Shopping List" below. This list shows you just how many fruits and vegetables you'll be enjoying on an all-you-can-eat basis. In this Appendix, you'll also discover some cooking tips, a variety of ways to spice up your fruits and veggies for more flavor, and you'll see which fruits and veggies rank highest in antioxident content.

The Overnight Diet Shopping List

Meat/Meat Substitutes
- ☐ Lean beef: London broil, top and bottom round, filet mignon
- ☐ Lean pork: pork chops, pork loin
- ☐ Fish: tuna steak, halibut, salmon, cod; or tuna, sardines, or salmon packed in water
- ☐ Poultry: skinless light meat chicken and turkey
- ☐ Eggs, egg whites, egg substitute
- ☐ Tofu, tempeh, or other soy products
- ☐ Meat alternatives

Protein
- ☐ Physicians Protein Smoothies Base Mix
- ☐ Casein protein
- ☐ Whey protein isolate

Milk and Milk Products

☐ Milk, fat-free, low-fat (1%)
☐ Dairy alternatives, fat-free, low-fat, unsweetened
☐ Cottage cheese, fat-free, low-fat (1%)
☐ Cheese, fat-free, low-fat
☐ Greek yogurt, fat-free, no fruit added
☐ Pudding, fat-free, sugar-free

Fruit

☐ Acai berries
☐ Apples
☐ Bananas
☐ Blackberries
☐ Blueberries
☐ Cantaloupe
☐ Cherimoyas
☐ Cherries
☐ Clementines
☐ Figs
☐ Grapefruit
☐ Grapes
☐ Guava
☐ Kiwis
☐ Lemons
☐ Limes
☐ Mangoes
☐ Marionberries
☐ Melons
☐ Nectarines
☐ Oranges
☐ Papayas
☐ Peaches
☐ Pears
☐ Persimmons
☐ Pineapple
☐ Plums
☐ Pomegranates
☐ Raspberries
☐ Star fruit
☐ Strawberries
☐ Watermelon
☐ Fruit canned in water or own juice, *not* syrup

Nonstarchy Vegetables

☐ Artichokes
☐ Asparagus
☐ Bamboo shoots
☐ Beans (green, wax, Italian)
☐ Bean sprouts
☐ Beets
☐ Bell peppers
☐ Broccoli
☐ Brussels sprouts
☐ Cabbage
☐ Carrots
☐ Cauliflower
☐ Celery
☐ Cucumbers
☐ Eggplant
☐ Greens (collard, mustard, turnip, Swiss chard)
☐ Kale
☐ Kohlrabi
☐ Leeks
☐ Lettuce
☐ Mushrooms
☐ Okra
☐ Onions
☐ Pea pods
☐ Rutabaga
☐ Sauerkraut
☐ Scallions
☐ Spinach
☐ Sprouts (alfalfa, mung bean, lentil)
☐ Summer squash
☐ Tomatoes
☐ Turnips
☐ Water chestnuts
☐ Zucchini

Starchy Vegetables/Legumes

- ☐ Black beans
- ☐ Black-eyed peas
- ☐ Cannellini
- ☐ Chickpeas (garbanzo beans)
- ☐ Corn
- ☐ Kidney beans
- ☐ Lentils
- ☐ Lima beans
- ☐ Navy beans
- ☐ Peas
- ☐ Pinto beans
- ☐ Potatoes
- ☐ Pumpkin
- ☐ Red beans
- ☐ Split peas
- ☐ Sweet potatoes
- ☐ White beans
- ☐ Winter squash
- ☐ Yams
- ☐ Yucca

Whole Grains

- ☐ Bagel, whole-grain
- ☐ Bread, whole-wheat
- ☐ Cold cereal, high-protein, high-fiber
- ☐ Couscous
- ☐ Farro
- ☐ Oatmeal
- ☐ Oat bran or cream of wheat cereal
- ☐ Pasta, whole-wheat
- ☐ Quinoa
- ☐ Rice, brown
- ☐ Crackers, whole-grain

Fats and Fat Alternatives

- ☐ Almonds
- ☐ Avocados
- ☐ Cashews
- ☐ Cooking spray, olive oil
- ☐ Cumin seeds
- ☐ Fennel seeds
- ☐ Flaxseeds
- ☐ Flaxseed oil
- ☐ Mayonnaise, fat-free, low-fat
- ☐ Olive oil
- ☐ Peanuts
- ☐ Peanut butter
- ☐ Pine nuts
- ☐ Pumpkin seeds
- ☐ Salad dressings, fat-free, low-fat
- ☐ Sesame seeds
- ☐ Sunflower seeds
- ☐ Walnuts

Sweets

- ☐ Artificial sweeteners (Truvia, Splenda)
- ☐ Chocolate chips
- ☐ Chocolate syrup, fat-free
- ☐ Cocoa powder, unsweetened
- ☐ Dried fruits
- ☐ Sugar-free hard candy
- ☐ Sugar-free Jell-O
- ☐ Sugar-free chewing gum

Condiments

☐ Basil

☐ Lemon juice

☐ Lime juice

☐ Mustard

☐ Onion powder

☐ Garlic powder

☐ Celery powder

☐ Oregano

☐ Pepper

☐ Salt

☐ Spices, flavorings, extracts

☐ Vinegar

Beverages

☐ Coffee

☐ Tea

☐ Water

☐ Seltzer water`

☐ Flavored water

☐ Tomato juice cocktail

☐ Sugar-free hot cocoa

☐ Juice (for smoothies only)

☐ Diet sodas (less than 2 calories)

The Overnight Diet Cooking Tips

The Overnight Diet meals are designed to be quick and easy to cook. In fact, some of them require no cooking at all. To make food preparation even easier, here are a few suggestions.

Sautéing. Use a nonstick cooking pan and extra virgin olive oil (not loads of butter) to sauté veggies. Sautéing means cooking at medium-high to high heat and stirring often. Extra virgin olive oil has heart-healthy benefits such as lowering cholesterol and improving insulin and blood sugar levels. Even so, it's a fat, which makes it high in calories. Use it sparingly or outfit your kitchen with the Misto Gourmet Olive Oil Sprayer or the Touch of Oil nonaerosol sprayer. They let you lightly spray, rather than glob, olive oil on cooking pans or on grilled or roasted veggies. You'll get all the flavor of heart-healthy extra virgin olive oil without all the extra fat and calories.

Add more veggies. Eat as many nonstarchy veggies as you'd like. Even if a recipe calls for 1 cup of spinach or 1 handful of spinach, feel free to throw in an extra handful, two handfuls, or even the whole bag.

Eggs, egg whites, and egg substitutes. Fresh whole eggs are a great source of protein and other nutrients. If you have heart disease or high cholesterol, stick to no more than seven whole eggs per week and opt for egg whites or liquid egg substitutes to make up the difference. Note that whole eggs, egg whites, and liquid egg substitutes differ in protein content. Check "How Much Protein Equals 1 Ounce of Protein Toward Your DPR" on page 71 for more information.

Poaching eggs. For perfectly poached eggs, place metal egg cups in a shallow pan of softly boiling water for 3–5 minutes or until the egg whites are done.

Keeping lean beef moist. Extra lean ground beef can sometimes be drier than the fattier versions. Adding vegetables, such as finely grated or puréed carrots, to burger patties and meatloaf helps lock moisture in for more juiciness.

Frozen versus fresh. It's okay to use either frozen or fresh fruits and vegetables on the Overnight Diet. However, you should be aware that frozen products are quicker to use, don't spoil as quickly as fresh, and often contain more nutrients because they are harvested at peak freshness.

Fat-free, low-fat, or dairy-free milk. Most of the recipes in this book call for fat-free milk, but you can also use 1% low-fat milk or any dairy-free milk of your choice, including soy milk, unsweetened almond milk, or light coconut milk.

Slicing avocados. Not sure how to tackle an avocado? With a sharp knife, score the outside lengthwise to the pit, and split into two halves. Whack the side of the pit with your knife and twist for easy removal. Wrap the unused half in plastic wrap to keep it from browning.

Preparing a pomegranate. If you want to toss some pomegranate seeds into a smoothie or a salad or you just want to snack on them, follow these simple steps. Cut off the top and bottom, then cut the fruit in half. Place it in a large bowl of cold water. Keep it underwater while you pick out the seeds. The seeds will sink to the bottom, and the rest will float to the top. Throw away the skin and white pithy part, then strain the seeds and enjoy.

Spice Up Your Veggies

Which herbs and spices go best with which vegetables?
Use this handy chart to find combinations you love.

Asparagus	Garlic, lemon juice, mustard seed, onion, paprika, parsley, tarragon, vinegar
Broccoli	Caraway seed, curry, dill, garlic, mustard seed, tarragon
Brussels sprouts	Basil, caraway seed, dill, garlic, mustard seed, sage, thyme
Cabbage	Caraway seed, celery seed, dill, mint, mustard seed, nutmeg, savory, tarragon
Carrots	Allspice, bay leaves, caraway seed, curry, dill, ginger, mace, marjoram, mint, nutmeg, parsley, thyme
Cauliflower	Caraway seed, curry, dill, garlic, mace, paprika, saffron, tarragon
Cucumber	Basil, chives, dill, garlic, mint, parsley, tarragon, vinegar
Eggplant	Marjoram, oregano
Green salads	Basil, chives, dill, parsley, tarragon
Green or wax beans	Basil, dill, garlic, lemon juice, marjoram, mint, mustard seed, nutmeg, oregano, paprika, parsley, savory, tarragon, thyme
Mushrooms	Garlic, oregano, paprika, pepper, saffron, sage
Onions	Caraway seed, chili pepper, cilantro, curry, garlic, mustard seed, nutmeg, oregano, paprika, saffron, sage, thyme
Spinach	Basil, garlic, mace, marjoram, nutmeg, oregano, saffron
Summer squash	Garlic, oregano, paprika, saffron, tarragon, basil
Tomatoes	Basil, bay leaves, celery seed, chili pepper, cilantro, garlic, marjoram, oregano, parsley, sage, tarragon, thyme
Zucchini	Basil, cilantro, garlic, oregano, paprika, parsley, saffron, tarragon

Spice Up Your Fruit

Herbs and spices that enhance the flavor of fruit

Chaat masala	Peppermint
Cinnamon	Poppy seeds
Clove	Spearmint
Coriander	Vanilla bean
Mint leaves	

Fruits and Vegetables High in Antioxidants

Acai berries	Kiwis
Beets	Oranges
Blackberries	Plums
Blueberries	Pomegranates
Broccoli	Raspberries
Brussels sprouts	Red bell peppers
Carrots	Red grapes
Cherries	Strawberries
Cranberries	Spinach
Kale	

Appendix C

25 Extra Delicious Smoothie Recipes

Because of the overwhelming positive response I received for my delicious and satisfying smoothies, I've added twenty-five smoothies to this edition—they are the most popular ones from my recipe book, *Diet Smoothies*. These smoothies are full of powerful protein, good-for-you wholesome fruits and vegetables, and healthy fiber. In this appendix, you will find recipes for "sinlessly" sumptuous smoothies, fruity smoothies that pack a flavorful punch, nutritious green smoothies bursting with thirst-quenching goodness, and simple smoothie recipes for those hectic workdays. Each and every recipe in this chapter makes a tasty and satisfying choice for breakfast, lunch, and dinner on your 1-Day Power Up, or a meal replacement during your 6-Day Fuel Up. As with my other smoothie recipes, feel free to make changes as you (and your taste buds) see fit. Just can't stomach a banana? Try substituting a small apple, a pear, or 1 cup of berries! Whether you choose to use fresh, frozen, or canned produce, you will lose weight with these heavenly delights.

To satisfy even the strongest sweet tooth, I've included my favorite recipes such as Crazy for Cocoa, Sweet Temptation, and Cherry Vanilla Apple Crumble. Are savory smoothies more your speed? Take the Kale Kickstart for a spin! If an easy and satisfying morning sipper is what you're after, start your day off right with The Grape Debate or Cheery Cherry. From cherries to berries and watercress to lettuce, each smoothie highlights the naturally delicious flavor of the bounty of fruits and vegetables found in each recipe.

These smoothies only *taste* decadent—each recipe contains a perfectly proportioned nutritive profile to ensure you're sipping your way slender!

Acai Action

Protein: 1 serving protein powder (Physicians Protein Smoothies Base Mix, or whey, or soy)

3 tablespoons acai berry juice

1 cup strawberries

½ cup blueberries

1 large banana

½–1 cup water

Ice (optional)

Power Berry

Protein: 1 serving protein powder (Physicians Protein Smoothies Base Mix, or whey, or soy)

3 tablespoons acai berry juice

1 large banana

1 cup seedless grapes

1 cup romaine lettuce

½ cup mint leaves

½–1 cup water

Ice (optional)

The Great Grapple

Protein: 1 serving protein powder (Physicians Protein Smoothies Base Mix, or whey, or soy)

1 large apple, peeled, cored, and chopped

1 cup seedless grapes

1 large carrot, peeled

2 cups Swiss chard

½–1 cup water

Ice (optional)

Banana-Nut Bread

Protein: 1 serving protein powder (Physicians Protein Smoothies Base Mix, or whey, or soy)

2 cups arugula

1 tablespoon creamy reduced-fat peanut butter

½ cup cinnamon-apple flavored tea (try Celestial Seasonings Cinnamon Apple)

½–1 cup water

Pinch of ground clove

Ice (optional)

Berry Delicious

Protein: 1 serving protein powder (Physicians Protein Smoothies Base Mix, or whey, or soy)

1 cup blackberries

½ cup raspberries

1 large banana

2 cups spinach

1 celery stalk

½–1 cup water

Ice (optional)

El Coco Canto

Protein: 1 serving protein powder (Physicians Protein Smoothies Base Mix, or whey, or soy)

1 cup cantaloupe

1 cup seedless grapes

2 cups spinach

1 cup coconut water

Ice (optional)

Sweet Temptation

Protein: 1 serving protein powder (Physicians Protein Smoothies Base Mix, or whey, or soy)

3 large carrots

1 cup mango

2 cups spinach

1 cup cucumber

1 teaspoon agave nectar (optional)

½–1 cup water

Ice (optional)

Cheery Cherry

Protein: 1 serving protein powder (Physicians Protein Smoothies Base Mix, or whey, or soy)

1 cup pitted cherries

1 large banana

2 cups spinach

½–1 cup water

Ice (optional)

Crazy for Cocoa

Protein: 1 serving protein powder (Physicians Protein Smoothies Base Mix, or whey, or soy)

1 cup strawberries

1 small orange, peeled and sectioned

2 cups romaine lettuce

2 tablespoons unsweetened cocoa powder

1 teaspoon agave nectar (optional)

½ cup fat-free milk

½ cup water

Ice (optional)

Coupe de Cucumber

Protein: 1 serving protein powder (Physicians Protein Smoothies Base Mix, or whey, or soy)

2 cups cucumber

2 cups cantaloupe

1 cup watermelon

1 ounce lemon juice

2 cups spinach

1 teaspoon agave nectar (optional)
½–1 cup water
Ice (optional)

Vitamin C Power Boost

Protein: 1 serving protein powder (Physicians Protein Smoothies Base Mix, or whey, or soy)
1 cup orange, peeled and sectioned
1 cup grapefruit, peeled and sectioned
1 cup fennel bulb, sliced
1 cup cucumber
Ice (optional)
½–1 cup water

Cherry Vanilla Apple Crumble

Protein: 1 serving protein powder (Physicians Protein Smoothies Base Mix, or whey, or soy)
1 cup pitted cherries
½ large apple, peeled, cored, and chopped
2 cups spinach
½ cup fat-free milk
½ cup water
1 tablespoon dry oats
½ teaspoon vanilla extract
Ice (optional)

FIGure Flatter

Protein: 1 serving protein powder (Physicians Protein Smoothies Base Mix, or whey, or soy)
3 small figs
1 large apple, peeled, cored, and chopped
1 large carrot, peeled
1 cup romaine lettuce
½–1 cup water
Ice (optional)

Juicebox Smoothie

Protein: 1 serving protein powder (Physicians Protein Smoothies Base Mix, or whey, or soy)

1 cup seedless grapes

½ cup blueberries

1 small tomato

2 cups spinach

1 large carrot

½–1 cup water

Ice (optional)

The Grape Debate

Protein: 1 serving protein powder (Physicians Protein Smoothies Base Mix, or whey, or soy)

1 cup seedless grapes

1 large banana

2 cups spinach

½–1 cup water

Ice (optional)

Orange Grango

Protein: 1 serving protein powder (Physicians Protein Smoothies Base Mix, or whey, or soy)

1 cup grapefruit

1 small orange, peeled and sectioned

½ cup mango

2 cups spinach

½–1 cup coconut water

Ice (optional)

Kale Kickstart

Protein: 1 serving protein powder (Physicians Protein Smoothies Base Mix, or whey, or soy)

1 cup kale

1 large banana

½ cup pineapple

1 small orange, peeled and sectioned

½–1 cup water

1 tablespoon grated ginger (optional)

Ice (optional)

Kwik Kiwi

Protein: 1 serving protein powder (Physicians Protein Smoothies Base Mix, or whey, or soy)

3 kiwis

1 cup strawberries

2 cups spinach

½–1 cup water

Ice (optional)

Strawberry Lemonade

Protein: 1 serving protein powder (Physicians Protein Smoothies Base Mix, or whey, or soy)

1 lemon, peeled, deseeded, and sectioned

1 large banana

1 cup strawberries

1 cup cucumber

1 cup spinach

½ teaspoon grated lemon zest (optional)

½–1 cup water

Ice (optional)

Much Ado About Mango

Protein: 1 serving protein powder (Physicians Protein Smoothies Base Mix, or whey, or soy)

1 cup mango

1 kiwi

2 cups romaine lettuce

1 cup coconut water

½ teaspoon almond extract (optional)

Ice (optional)

Oranga-Tang Apple

Protein: 1 serving protein powder (Physicians Protein Smoothies Base Mix, or whey, or soy)

1 cup pineapple

2 small oranges, peeled, deseeded, and sectioned

2 cups Swiss chard

2 celery stalks

½–1 cup water

½ teaspoon grated orange zest (optional)

Ice (optional)

Straw-Berry Explosion

Protein: 1 serving protein powder (Physicians Protein Smoothies Base Mix, or whey, or soy)

1 cup strawberries

½ cup blueberries

½ cup raspberries

½ large banana

2 cups romaine lettuce

1 small carrot

½–1 cup water

Ice (optional)

Watermelon Mojito

Protein: 1 serving protein powder (Physicians Protein Smoothies Base Mix, or whey, or soy)

2 cups seedless watermelon

1 ounce lime juice

½ cup mint leaves

1 cup strawberries

1 cup sliced cucumber

1 cup Italian parsley

½–1 cup water

Ice (optional)

Chocolate Monkey Shake

Protein: 1 serving protein powder (Physicians Protein Smoothies Base Mix, or whey, or soy)

1 small-sized banana

2 tablespoons unsweetened cocoa powder

1 cup fresh spinach

1 cup unsweetened almond milk

1 teaspoon flaxseeds (optional)

Ice (optional)

Lose the Water Weight Watercress

Protein: 1 serving protein powder (Physicians Protein Smoothies Base Mix, or whey, or soy)

1 apple, peeled, cored, and chopped

2 limes

1 cup watercress

2 whole carrots

2 celery stalks

1 cup sliced cucumber

½–1 cup water

Ice (optional)

Index

About the Authors

Dr. Caroline Apovian

In college, Caroline Apovian, MD, gained the Freshman 10, and then went on to achieve the Sophomore 15, and the Junior 20, before developing the seeds of this plan to help her slim down and shape up. Based on her own success, she wanted to share what she had learned. Helping others safely achieve rapid weight loss that lasts became her life's mission. For over twenty-five years, Dr. Apovian has held a position at the forefront of the obesity and weight-management field. One of the world's premier weight-loss experts, she has distinguished herself as a leading researcher, treatment provider, and teacher in the fields of obesity and weight loss while also working as director of the Nutrition and Weight Management Center at the Boston University Medical Center, co-director of the Nutrition and Metabolic Support Services at the Boston University Medical Center, director of Clinical Research at the Obesity Research Center of Boston University Medical Center, and professor of Medicine at Boston University School of Medicine.

Her federal government positions include nutrition consultant to NASA and appointed member of the federal government's panel on the evaluation and treatment of overweight adults.

Her unparalleled accomplishments in the obesity and weight-loss field, which have earned her recognition from her peers and made her a media favorite, include her popular weight-loss column on EverydayHealth.com; the Physician Nutrition Specialist Award presented by the American Society of Clinical Nutrition for advancing nutrition education among doctors and medical students; grants from diverse sources, ranging from the NIH to the Atkins Foundation to the Global Health Primary Care Initiative; and television appearances from *The Dr. Oz Show* to the Discovery Channel.

A frequent national and international lecturer, Dr. Apovian has published papers, reviews, and book chapters on nutrition, obesity, and nutrition support and serves as manuscript reviewer for several prestigious journals, including: *New England Journal of Medicine, Journal of Women's Health, International Journal of Obesity, Obesity Research, Digestive and Liver Disease,* and *Journal of Parenteral and Enteral Nutrition.*

Her editorial positions have included: *International Journal of Food Safety, Nutrition and Public Health* (associate editor), *BMC Research Notes* (associate editor), *Current Opinion in Endocrinology and Diabetes* (editor of the Nutrition and Obesity section), *Obesity* (associate editor), *Nutrition in Clinical Practice* (associate editor), and *American Journal of Clinical Nutrition* (guest science editor). Her professional activities also include serving as chair of the Obesity Research Interest Section for the American Society for Nutrition, principal investigator for the Center for Obesity Research and Education, executive committee member of the Boston Nutrition Obesity Research Center, member of the Task Force on Physician Credentialing in the Obesity Medicine Subspecialty, director of the Nutrition Support Fellowship, director of the Nutrition and Obesity Medicine Fellowship, and associate director of the Graduate Program in Medical Nutrition Sciences.

Dr. Caroline Apovian lives in Waban, Massachusetts, with her husband and two sons. Her website is www.OvernightDiet.org and her Facebook page is www.facebook/dr.caroline.apovian.

Diana Cullum-Dugan

Diana Cullum-Dugan, RD, LD RYT, is a licensed dietician nutritionist as well as a registered yoga teacher who began working with Dr. Apovian in 1999. As a plump twelve-year-old with overweight aunts, Diana recognized a strong familial tendency to gain weight.

To combat her predisposition, her parents sent her to a health spa, setting her on her career path of helping people interested in weight loss. At Boston Medical Center, Diana managed the outpatient Nutrition and Weight Management Center and multiple clinical nutrition trials. At the same institution, she was the lead yoga teacher in a study of Yoga for Low Back Pain and is the exercise and nutrition expert of a respected web-based nutrition/exercise intervention program.

Diana regularly lectures on weight management and nutritional assessment to wide audiences at Harvard University Medical School, Boston University's Sargent College, Northwest University School of Medicine, and the American Dietetic Association.

Wayne L. Westcott

Wayne L. Westcott, PhD, directed fitness research programs at the South Shore YMCA in Quincy, Massachusetts, for more than twenty-five years. Wayne has been a strength-training consultant for numerous organizations, including the United States Navy, the American Council on Exercise, and the YMCA of the USA. He has authored or coauthored twenty-four books and textbooks and more than sixty peer-reviewed papers. Wayne serves as an editorial advisor, reviewer, writer, and columnist for many publications, including *Prevention, Shape, The Physician and Sportsmedicine,* and ACSM's *Health & Fitness Journal.* He has been the keynote speaker for national meetings of the American College of Sports Medicine, the American College of Nutrition, and the National Intramural and Recreational Sports Association. Wayne has served on the executive committee for the New England Chapter of the American College of Sports Medicine, as well as on the advisory boards for the International Council on Active Aging and the International Association of Fitness Professionals. He has received the Lifetime Achievement Award from the International Association of Fitness Professionals and the Healthy American Fitness Leader Award from the President's Council on Physical Fitness and Sports.

Frances Sharpe

Frances Sharpe is a writer and ghostwriter who has been covering health and wellness, fitness, and diet for nearly twenty years. She is the ghostwriter of two *New York Times* bestsellers as well as seventeen other well-received nonfiction books. Her work has also appeared in *The Huffington Post, AARP—The Magazine, Entrepreneur, Health, Women's Health & Fitness, Muscle & Body Magazine, WellBella Magazine, Teen People,* and on Playboy.com.